10 Steps to a New You

Or

The 10 Little Known Steps to Lose Weight in 60 Days or Less
& Keep it Off Forever – without Dieting

By Susie Ellis

This is NOT a Diet

This is all about making a few small sustainable changes that will help you feel pleased with yourself & then you will be comfortable with taking another small positive step.
It is called the compound effect!

Broadly the ten steps are:
- Your own body shape
- Hunger
- Habit or addiction?
- Stress factors & illness; cause & prevention
- Hypothalamus & chewing
- Water
- Salt
- Butter & oil v spread
- Confidence
- Movement & exercise

Contents:

Part I

Achievable targets
Compound effect
History & the Diet Industry
Love your Body
Homework

This is Not a Diet

Anything we do for 21 days becomes a habit.... so baby steps

We are going to set ourselves some achievable targets
...compound effect

Current thinking & research tells us, that people gain weight
for a great of variety reasons & there are a vast number of
businesses & 'experts' making money out of exploiting the
situation.

This is different. I want to help you be happier, healthier &
have more self esteem by achieving your ideal body weight
& image. No more yo-yo dieting; no more bingeing &
starving - this is a lifestyle challenge so stick with it & it will
last forever.

There is no 'one size fits all' solution & unfortunately I don't
have a magic wand so we are going to have to discover why
you are carrying extra weight so that you will be able to
make some life changing decisions for yourself...

One Step at a Time

I'm going to take you through a simple step-by-step process
to kick start your journey to the new you.

We're going to examine all the downsides; why people gain
weight, why that is an unhealthy state to be in, the illnesses
that are caused by obesity ...
& we are going to examine all the upsides... what your life
will be like when you achieve your goal weight, what you
will be able to do that you can't do now, how proud your
family & friends will be of your success... & of course your
self esteem will sky rocket

This is going to be an ongoing journey; a true life
turnaround & I'm going to help you every step of the way.

History

Let's go back in time.....World War II 1939 - 1945 Rationing
Weekly rations varied in the UK from month to month as
foods became more or less plentiful & continued until 1954.
In 1946 bread was rationed & the sweet ration was halved

Typical ration for 1 adult per week:-
- Butter: 50g (2oz)
- Sugar: 225g (8oz)
- Cheese: 2oz (50g)
- Jam: 450g (1lb) every two months
- Meat: To the value of 1s 6d [7 ½ p] or $0.53
  [today £7.12 or $11.38]
- Bacon and ham: 100g (4oz)
- Eggs: 1 fresh egg a week
- Dried eggs 1 packet every four weeks
- Margarine: 100g (4oz)
- Tea: 50g (2oz)
- Milk: 3 pints (1800ml) occasionally dropping
  to 2 pints (1200ml)
- Sweets: 350g (12oz) every four weeks [87.5 g /
  3ozs per week]

Other rationed foods include fish, rice, dried fruit, tin
tomatoes, tinned peas, biscuits, sausages, canned fruit,
breakfast cereals, milk & cooking fat

There was also a points system which limited the purchase of tinned or imported goods. 16 points in the ration book were available every 4 weeks to purchase something different... 1 can of tinned fish or 2lbs of dried fruit or 8 lbs of split peas

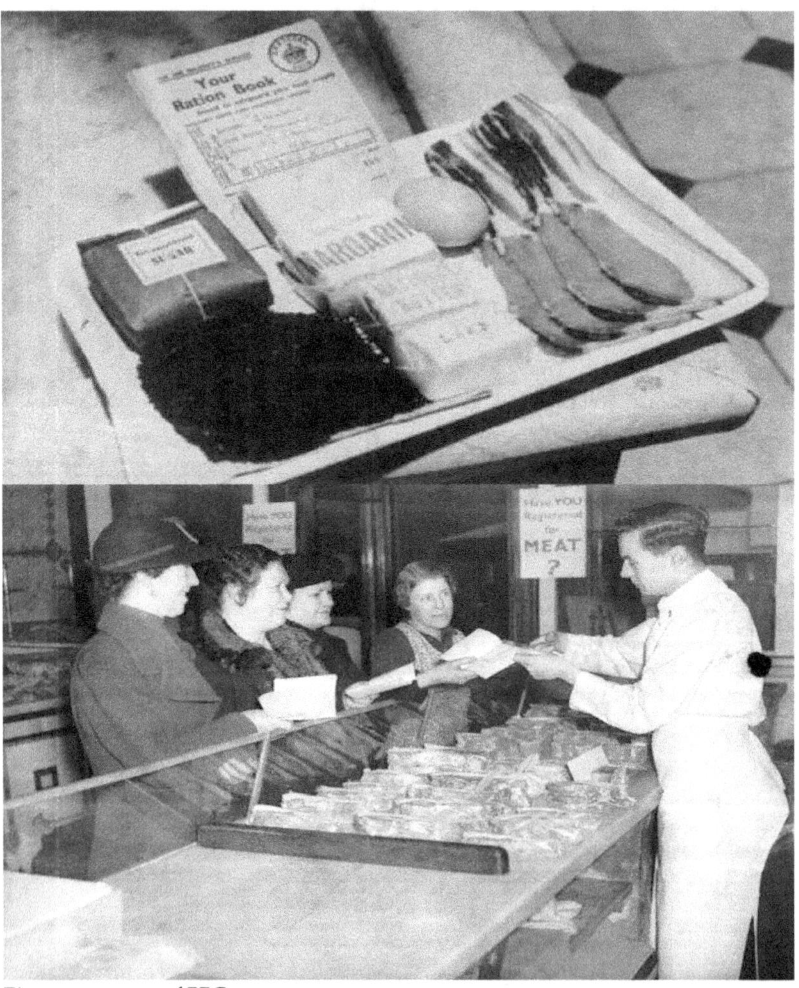

Pictures courtesy of BBC

Feb. 1, 1944
SPECIAL NOTE:
Token program begins Feb. 27.
One-point red tokens will be given
in change for Red Stamps and one-
point Blue Tokens for Blue
Stamps. Stamps will be worth 10
points each. Tear Stamps out
cross Ration Book instead of up
and down. Following Stamps be-
come valid Feb. 27:
MEATS AND FATS
Red Stamps A8, B8 and C8
(Book Four) good for 10 points
each, Feb. 27 through Ma_ 20.
PROCESSED FOODS
Blue Stamps A8, B8, C8, D8
(Book Four) good for 10 points
each, Feb. 27 through May 20.
Following Stamps remain at pres-
sent point values.
PROCESSED FOODS
Green Stamps G, H and J (Book
Four) good Jan. 1 through Feb. 20.
Green Stamps K, L and M (Book
Four) good Feb. 1 through Mar. 20
MEATS AND FATS
Brown Stamps V (Book Three)
good Jan. 23 through Feb. 26.
Brown Stamps W good Jan. 30
through Feb. 26.
Brown Stamps X good Feb. 6
through Feb. 26.
Brown Stamps Y good Feb. 13
through Mar. 20.
Brown Stamps Z good Feb. 20
through Mar 20.
SUGAR
Stamp No. 30 (Book Four) good
for five pounds Jan. 16 through
Mar. 31.
SHOES
Stamp No. 18 (Book One) good
for one pair indefinitely. Airplane
Stamp No. 1 (Book Three) good
for one pair indefinitely.
FUEL OIL
Period No. 2 coupons good for
ten gallons per unit through Feb.
7.
Period No. 3 coupons good for
ten gallons per unit through Mar.
13.
Period No. 4 coupons and Period
No. 5 coupons good for ten gallons
per unit Feb. 8 th ough Sept. 30.
GASOLINE
No. 10 coupons in A book good
for three gallons each Jan. 22
through Mar. 21.
B2 and C2 supplemental ration
coupons good for five gallons each.
B1 and C1 coupons remain good
for two gallons each. All coupons

Why am I telling you this? Because people didn't go hungry
& they weren't overweight!

However by 2014 in the UK 64% [BBC] & in the USA 66% [Ogden
et al] of people are overweight or obese

In 1972 when British scientist John Yudkin first proved that sugar was bad for our health, he was ignored by the majority of the medical profession and rubbished by the food industry.   When I quoted from his book 'Pure White & Deadly' people thought I was being daft.
[see https://ww.susieellis.org/recommended-reading/]

Have a look on the web there are plenty of videos showing that sugar is as addictive as cocaine.

Plus there seems to be a link in the incidences of bowel related diseases in those people old enough to have lived on 'rations' & then devoured the 'pure white & deadly' foods

Diet Industry

The Diet Industry is big business. As obesity became a problem more & more companies saw the chance to make money & jumped on the band wagon.

There are slimming clubs which have brought out their own replacement food products; there are companies selling meal replacement shakes and snacks & much more.

Please be aware that you are being sold to. Every time there is a TV advert or you see a picture in a magazine remember that they are concerned about gaining customers for their business; you buying their product is important to their financial balance sheet. It is estimated that 80% of the 'foods' on supermarket shelves didn't exist 100 years ago.

In 2002 Eric Schlosser published the book 'Fast Food Nation' proving that chemicals are added to many 'fast foods' that switch off the hypothalamus so the consumer never feels full & others that create addiction.
[see https://ww.susieellis.org/recommended-reading/]

This might look like a comic but it is deadly serious...

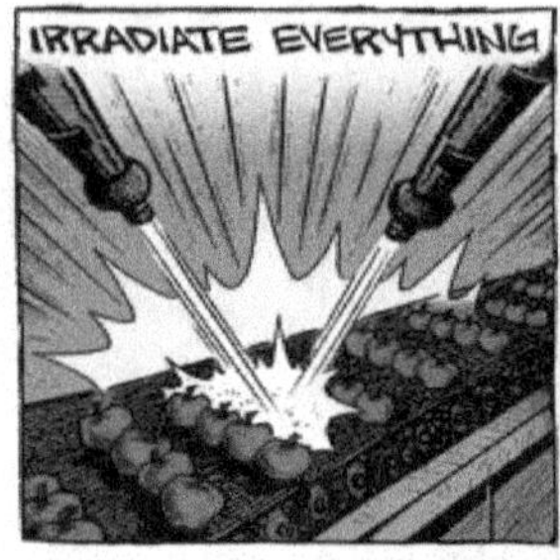
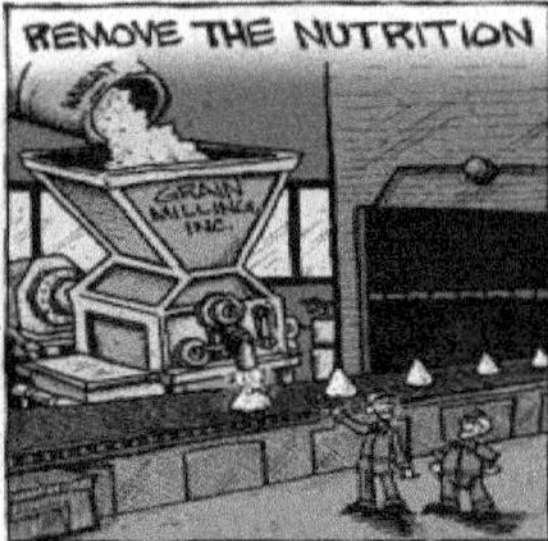
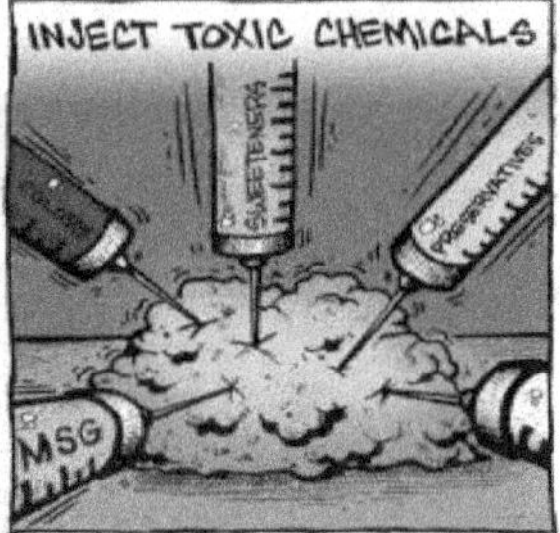
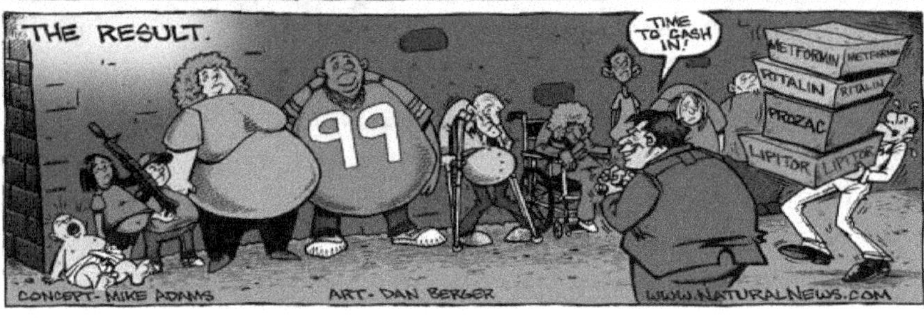

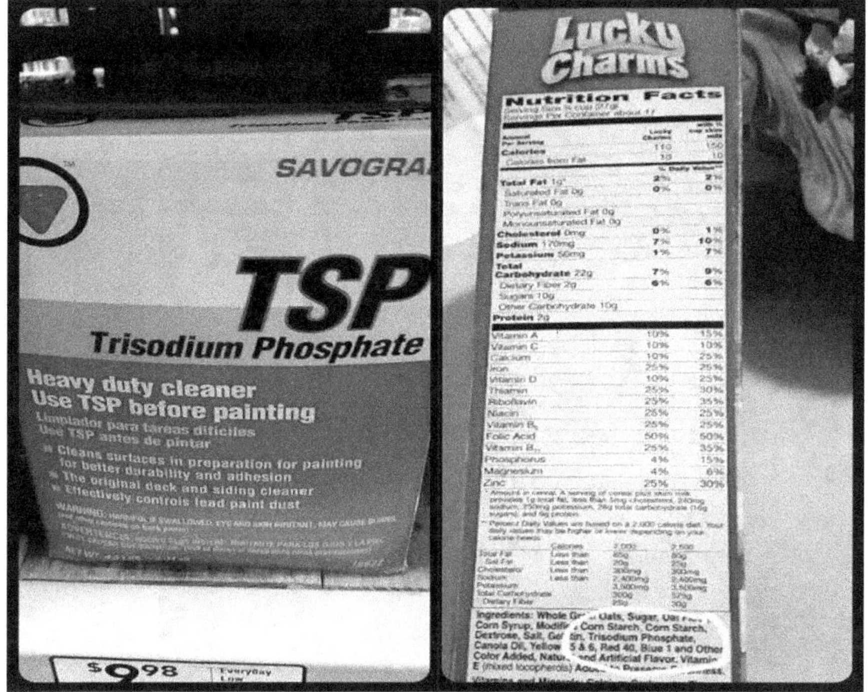

Photo Courtesy of NewWorldOutlawzKilluminati

Read every packet in your kitchen cupboards & become aware of the stuff you are ingesting that isn't food. I'm not suggesting that you throw out everything in a packet but do try, when stuff runs out, to replace it with a healthier alternative.

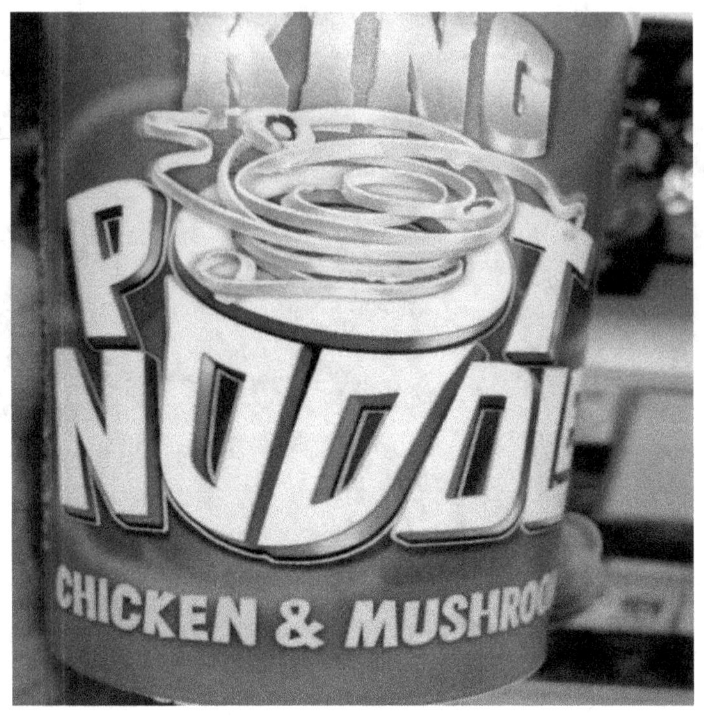

The title suggests chicken but as you can clearly see on the next page in the ingredients list…there isn't any!

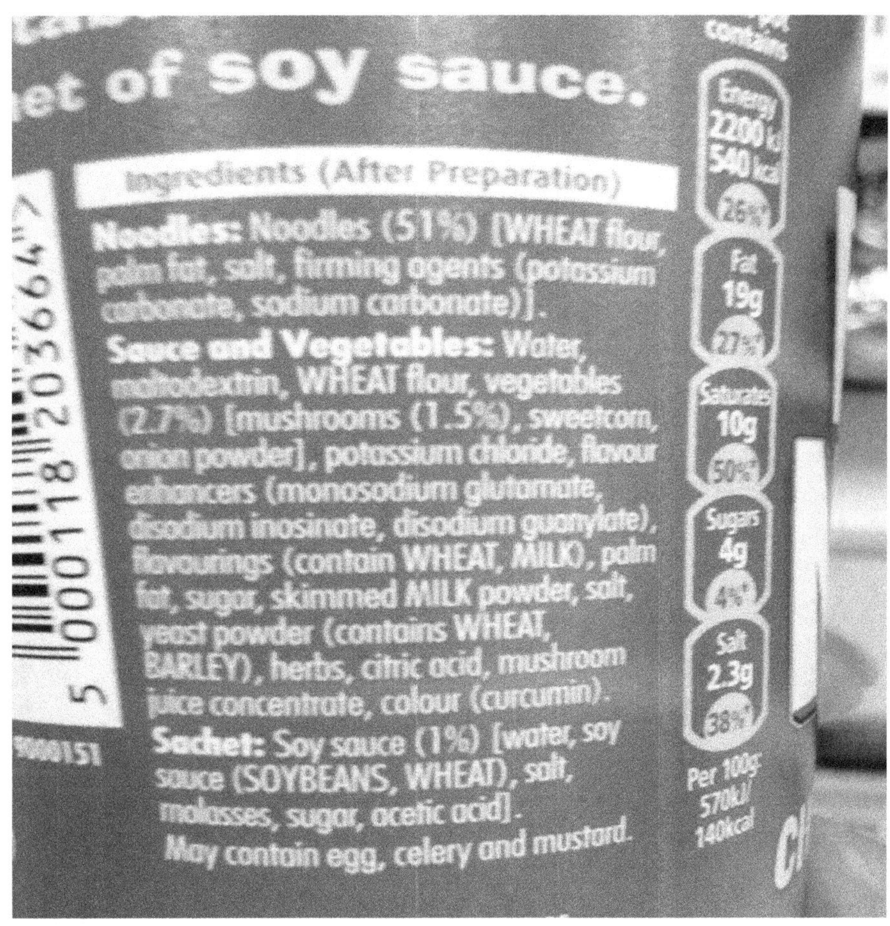

I've written a recipe for you so you can quickly make your own healthy Pot Noodle

... you can find it in Part III

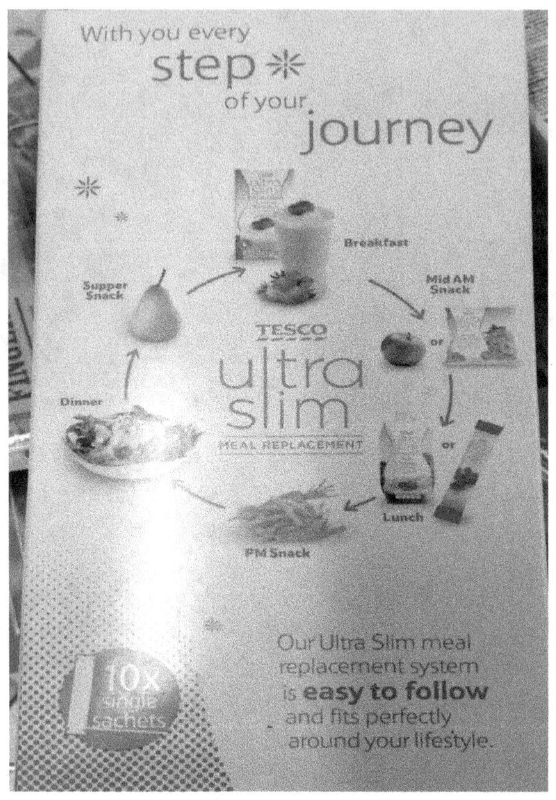

This will provide approx 200 kcal per serving using 29g powder made up with 250 ml skimmed milk ~

but take a look at the ingredients on the next page…

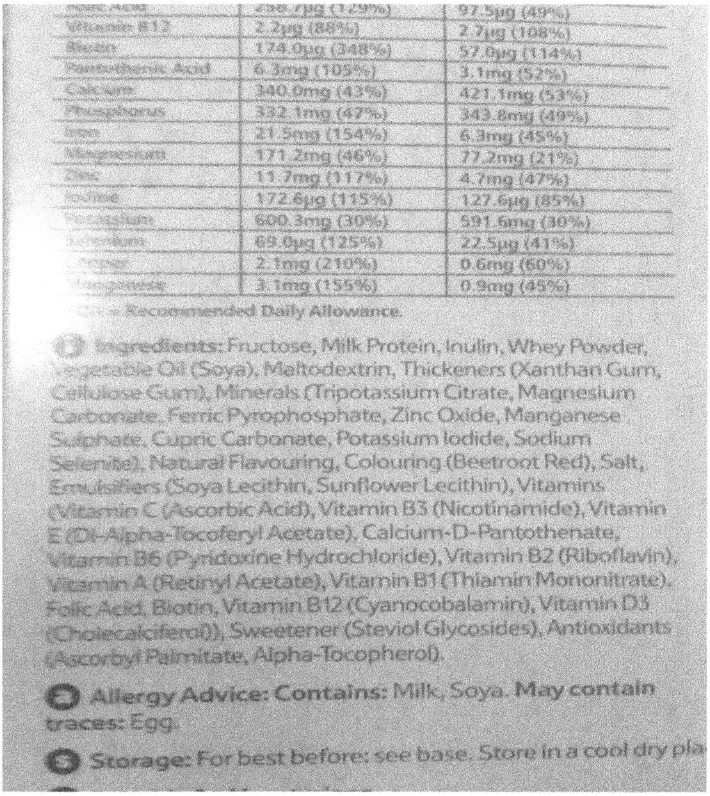

Folic Acid	258.7µg (129%)	97.5µg (49%)
Vitamin B12	2.2µg (88%)	2.7µg (108%)
Biotin	174.0µg (348%)	57.0µg (114%)
Pantothenic Acid	6.3mg (105%)	3.1mg (52%)
Calcium	340.0mg (43%)	421.1mg (53%)
Phosphorus	332.1mg (47%)	343.8mg (49%)
Iron	21.5mg (154%)	6.3mg (45%)
Magnesium	171.2mg (46%)	77.2mg (21%)
Zinc	11.7mg (117%)	4.7mg (47%)
Iodine	172.6µg (115%)	127.6µg (85%)
Potassium	600.3mg (30%)	591.6mg (30%)
Selenium	69.0µg (125%)	22.5µg (41%)
Copper	2.1mg (210%)	0.6mg (60%)
Manganese	3.1mg (155%)	0.9mg (45%)

* = Recommended Daily Allowance.

Ingredients: Fructose, Milk Protein, Inulin, Whey Powder, Vegetable Oil (Soya), Maltodextrin, Thickeners (Xanthan Gum, Cellulose Gum), Minerals (Tripotassium Citrate, Magnesium Carbonate, Ferric Pyrophosphate, Zinc Oxide, Manganese Sulphate, Cupric Carbonate, Potassium Iodide, Sodium Selenite), Natural Flavouring, Colouring (Beetroot Red), Salt, Emulsifiers (Soya Lecithin, Sunflower Lecithin), Vitamins (Vitamin C (Ascorbic Acid), Vitamin B3 (Nicotinamide), Vitamin E (DI-Alpha-Tocoferyl Acetate), Calcium-D-Pantothenate, Vitamin B6 (Pyridoxine Hydrochloride), Vitamin B2 (Riboflavin), Vitamin A (Retinyl Acetate), Vitamin B1 (Thiamin Mononitrate), Folic Acid, Biotin, Vitamin B12 (Cyanocobalamin), Vitamin D3 (Cholecalciferol)), Sweetener (Steviol Glycosides), Antioxidants (Ascorbyl Palmitate, Alpha-Tocopherol).

Allergy Advice: Contains: Milk, Soya. May contain traces: Egg.

Storage: For best before: see base. Store in a cool dry pla

Just look at this meal replacement... why would you eat all those 'additives' when you could eat a jacket potato & baked beans for 200 kcal?

ultra
slim
SNACKS
Cheese
& Onion
OYA & POTATO SNACK
o artificial flavours,
lours or preservatives
Less than
99kcal
in this bag
Each serving contains
Calories
90
5%
Sugars
0.8g
1%
Fat
1.9g
3%
Satura
0.2
1%

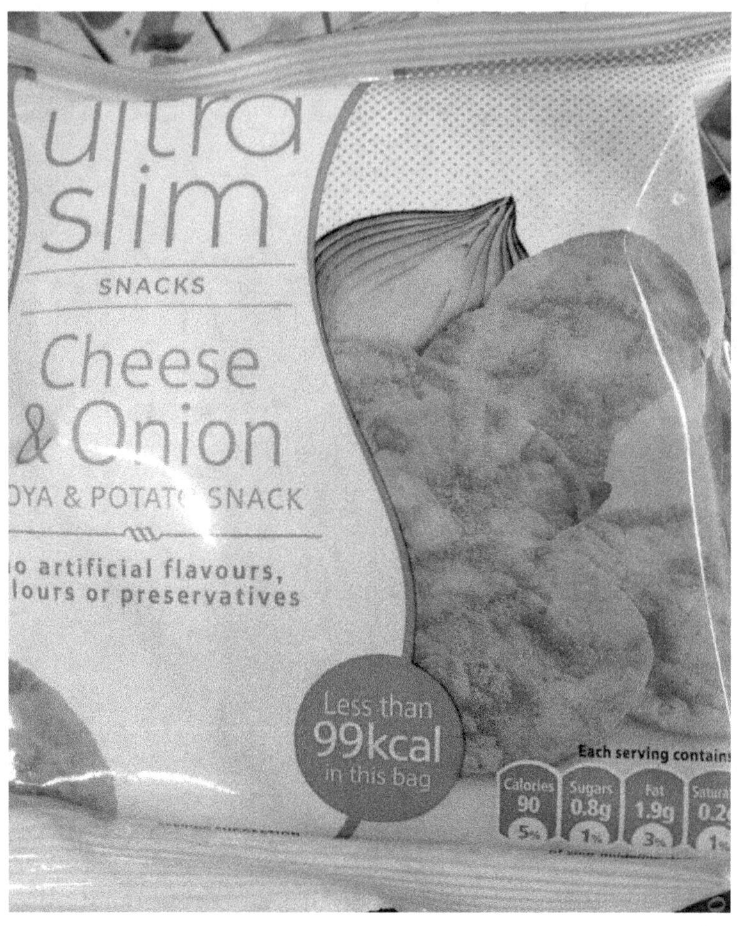

99 kcal!

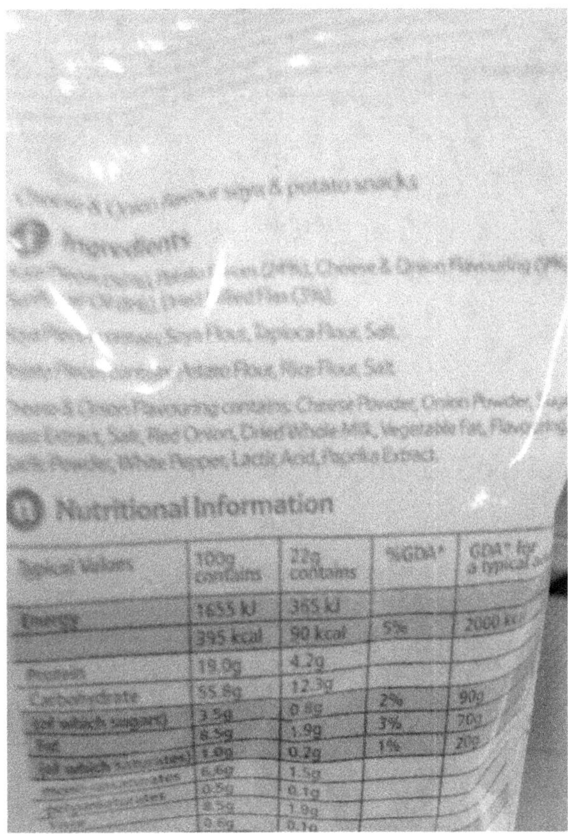

Why not replace these 'diet' snacks with 4 biscuits or a banana & a cup of tea!!! ?

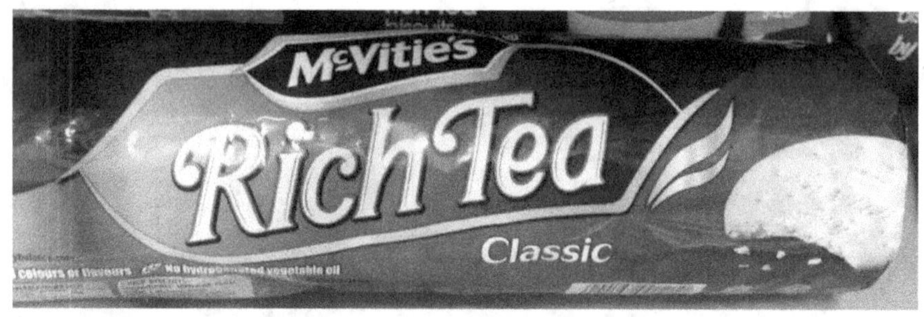

Do go & read the labels in your supermarket ... I am sure you can find some real food to replace your 'diet' products

Nutrition Information

ERAGE LUES	PER 100g	PER BISCUIT (8.3g)
RGY (kJ)	1929	160
(kcal)	459	38
	15.5g	1.3g
vhich SATURATES	1.5g	0.1g
BOHYDRATE	71.3g	5.9g
vhich SUGARS	20.2g	1.7g
RE	2.9g	0.2g
OTEIN	7.0g	0.6g
T	0.8g	0.1g

ical number of biscuits per pack: 36

CRISP BISCUITS
Ingredients: **Wheat** Flour (with Calcium, Iron, Niacin, Thiamin), Sugar, Vegetable Oil (Sunflower), Glucose-Fructose Syrup, **Barley** Malt Extract, Raising Agents (Sodium Bicarbonate, Ammonium Bicarbonate), Salt.

For allergens, including cereals containing gluten, see ingredients in **bold**. May also contain Soya.

Only 38 kcal per biscuit...

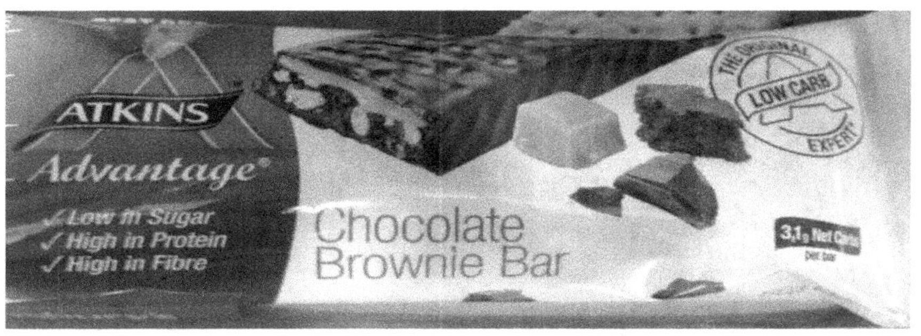

Values	Typische waarden	Valeurs Typiques	per 60 g	per 100 g
	Energie	Énergie	907 kJ	1511 kJ
			218 kcal	363 kcal
	Vet	Graisses	9,3 g	16 g
saturates	waarvan verzadigd	dont saturés	4,9 g	8,2 g
ate	Koolhydraten	Glucides	15,7 g	26,2 g
sugars	waarvan suikers	dont sucres	1,1 g	1,8 g
polyols	waarvan polyolen	dont polyols	12,6 g	21 g
	Voedingsvezels	Fibres alimentaires	9,4 g	16 g
	Eiwit	Protéines	18 g	30 g
	Zout	Sel	0,44 g	0,73 g

In this diet bar there are 218 kcal, a load of chemicals & a warning that it has a laxative effect, not pleasant.

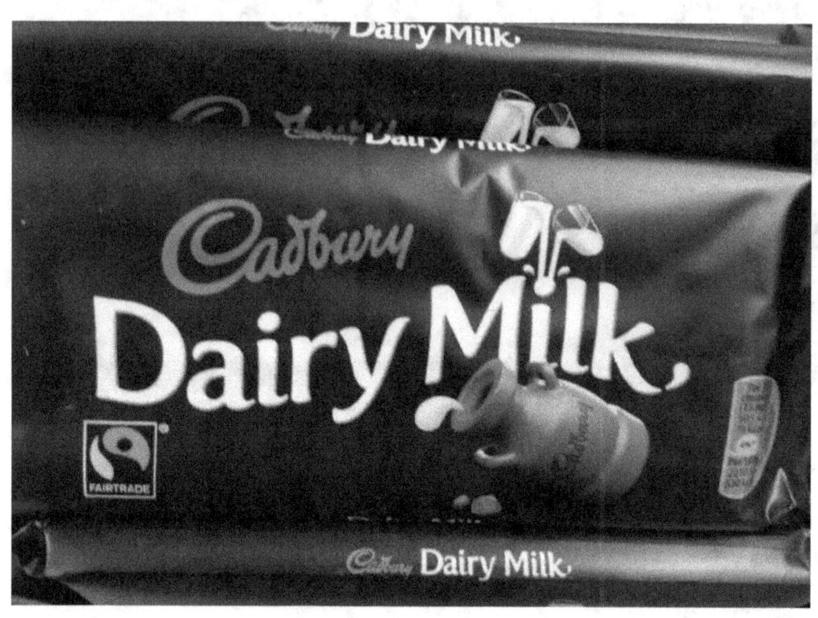

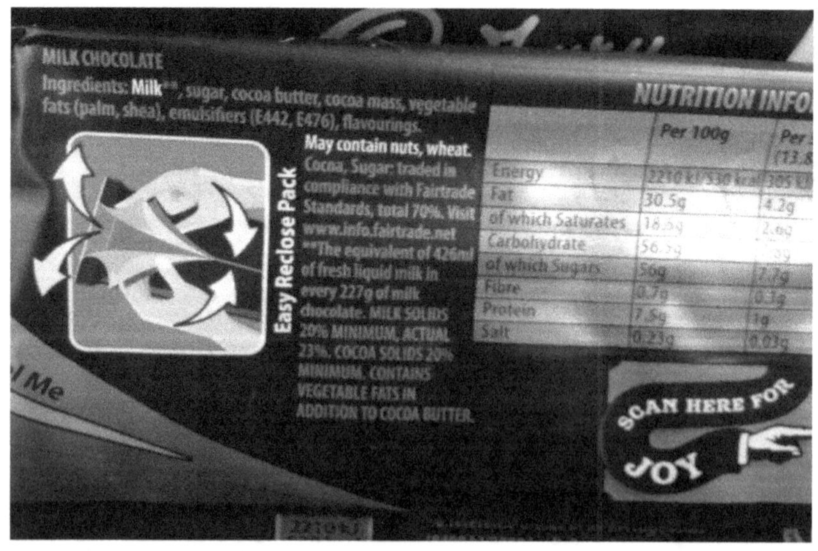

NUTRITION INFO	Per 100g	Per (13.8
Energy	2210 kJ/530 kcal	305 k
Fat	30.5g	4.2g
of which Saturates	18.5g	2.6g
Carbohydrate	56.5g	3g
of which Sugars	56g	7.7g
Fibre	0.7g	0.1g
Protein	7.5g	1g
Salt	0.23g	0.03g

People stared curiously whilst I photographed all of these products in my local supermarket but maybe it made a couple of people wonder what I was doing & start to read the backs of packets.

It is much better for your body to eat real food as that is what it recognises and can therefore digest & assimilate

Whatever you put in your mouth make sure you **truly enjoy & savour** every mouthful, no feeling guilty or naughty

.

Love Your Body

Go & stand in front of a full length mirror...
What would just 8lbs less look like?
Or maybe an inch off your waistline?
Make a first, achievable, initial goal

Which body shape are you?

Ectomorphs may not put on weight easily but they are subject to the same food related diseases.

Mesomorph & Endomorph body shapes are more prone to gaining excess weight but you need to learn to love your body, it's the only one you've got!

Be realistic about your goals

& Smile at yourself

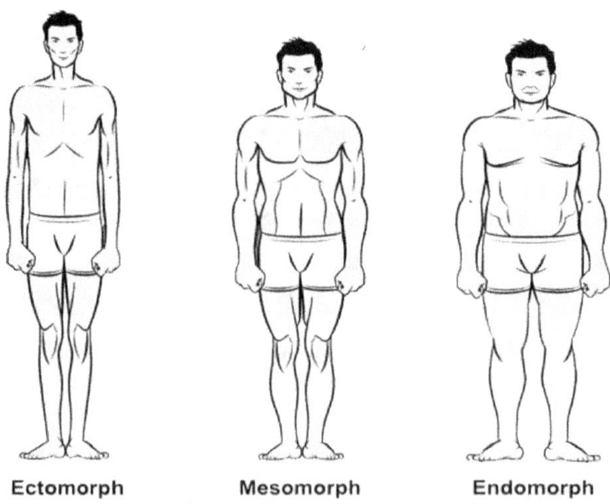

Courtesy of Govt of Western Aust Dept of Health

Homework

So here are your first 'baby steps'...

The idea is that you begin to make some small changes to the way you view yourself, your attitude towards your body and the food you eat. Every small change that you sustain gives you confidence. That confidence increases and gives you the incentive to do more; it is a compound effect.

- Look in a full length mirror, take note of how you feel and decide what small change would make the most difference. It may be an inch off your waist, toning up your stomach muscles... Just one small change to concentrate on first. Measure your waist or weigh yourself now & then put the scales & tape measure away for at least 60 days.

- Make a dream board, [mind map/screensaver/scrapbook] which includes a picture of you at your happy weight & pin it up in the kitchen

- Write down everything you put in your mouth that isn't a meal. Keep a notebook in the kitchen. As you go to eat something that isn't a meal ask yourself 'is this habit or is this addiction'? This concentrates your mind and you may think about putting it down &

having it later or thinking that you don't actually
need it. After a week you will be able to see how
much you eat that you were totally unaware of eating
& you will also be able to pinpoint the 'crisis' triggers.

Remember the compound effect...there is no rush!
Just do one thing at a time; turn one change into a new habit
& then add the next one.
Go at your own pace & learn to feel great about your
achievements.

Part II

Illness & Obesity
Insulin & Metabolism
Sugar addiction
Yo-yo dieting
Stress factors
Control by the media
Homework

This is not a diet

Now we are going to be looking at stress factors, the illnesses linked to obesity & what we can do to prevent them.

You might think this a bit doom & gloom but we do need to acknowledge the links between what goes into our bodies and the resulting effects. Once we understand the connections we can begin to take action and make some positive changes.

If you are going through a particularly stressful time be kind to yourself; just take in all this information & take action later when you are in a calmer state of mind. People sometimes just overdo things... They give up smoking, cut out alcohol, go on a diet & join a gym all at the same time...this is just too much all at once... & bound to fail

Make a few small sustainable changes; feel pleased with yourself & then you will be comfortable with taking another small positive step. The compound effect again!

Illness & Obesity

If you are overweight or obese, you are more prone to develop potentially serious health problems; according to the Mayo Clinic these include:

High triglycerides and low high-density lipoprotein (HDL) cholesterol
Type 2 diabetes, High blood pressure,
Metabolic syndrome — a combination of high blood sugar, high blood pressure, high triglycerides and low HDL cholesterol
Heart disease, Stroke, Cancer,
Breathing disorders, including sleep apnoea,
Gallbladder disease, Gynaecological problems, e.g. infertility & irregular periods
Erectile dysfunction
Non-alcoholic fatty liver disease, [fat builds up in the liver causing inflammation or scarring]
Osteoarthritis
Skin conditions, including poor wound healing

Insulin & Metabolism

The body uses three main fuels, glucose from sugar & carbohydrates, amino acids from proteins, and fatty acids from fats.

Insulin is a hormone which makes our body cells absorb glucose from the blood. Glucose is stored in the liver and muscles as glycogen which prevents the body using fat as a source of energy. If there is too little insulin in the blood, glucose is not taken up by our body cells & our body utilises fat as a source of energy.

Glucose provides energy for immediate needs but while you are eating the energy requirements are fulfilled so the extra energy must be stored for the future. One storage place is the liver, but storage space is limited & the other, with almost unlimited storage space, are the fat cells. Not what we want!

Diabetes is one illness caused by insulin production being disrupted; but the good news is that if we restrict sugar to the amount the body can actually utilise balance is restored.

Sugar addiction

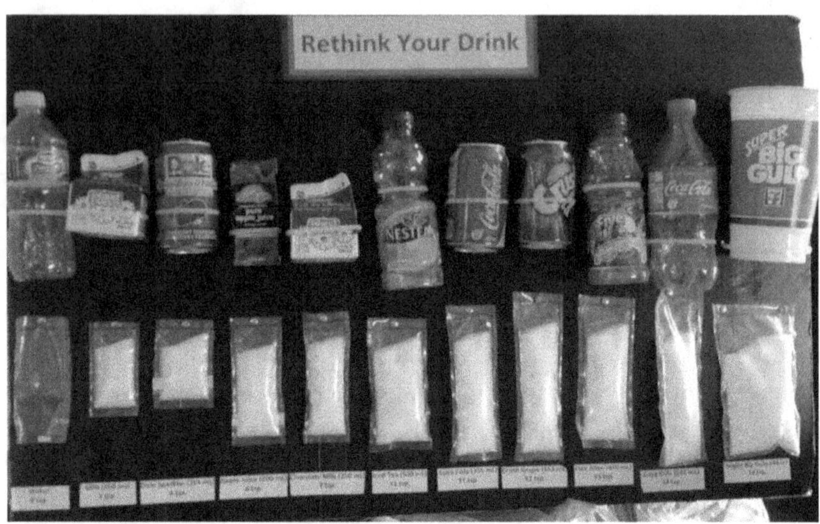

Photo Courtesy of Sustain our Africa

This is a photograph of a school project to illustrate exactly how much sugar is in each drink

Sugar has been found to be as addictive as cocaine so if you can kick this habit you will be giving yourself the best start to repairing damage.

More about this in Part V

YoYo Dieting

Why, when you go first go on a diet do you lose weight but when you stop dieting you put the weight back on & often gain even more?

It is estimated that 54% of people in the US are trying to lose weight & that a dieter will try a new plan four times a year…. Weight cycling, as experts call it, repeated dieting, raises hormone levels which in turn causes you to start putting weight on around your midriff. Research has linked this cycle to diabetes, high blood pressure and heart disease.

So why does this happen? When you go on a diet & eat fewer calories or fewer carbohydrates, your body goes into famine response. You lose weight from your lean muscle and fluids because your blood sugar drops, your metabolic rate slows down & hormone glucagon is released which burns body muscle. There is an increase in fat storage in your cells. You get fed up with being hungry & miserable & develop cravings. Then you start eating normally again or over-eat or re introduce carbohydrates. This is called the feast response where you eat more calories than you need & you regain more fat. Then as the hormone insulin is released your blood sugar spikes which leads to weight & body fat increase.

A vicious circle…. which we can break…

Stress

Food stress is probably the first thing to tackle & I have talked about this before. If your body doesn't understand what you are putting in it i.e. chemicals & not food, then it become stressed. If you eat food created by men in white coats then you are going to end up being treated by men in white coats!

Another stress when you are overweight is that your quality of life might be lower. You may not be able to do things you'd like to or participate in some activities which may lead to you feeling depressed & isolated

But it might just be that you have over ambitious goals... so let's bust some myths...

Don't Believe Everything...

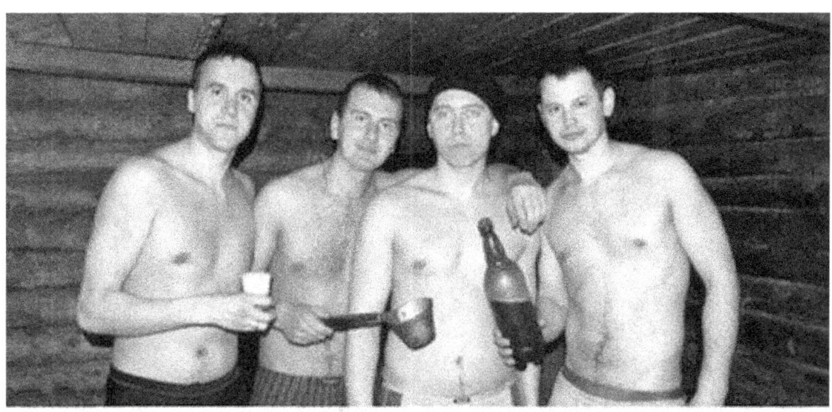

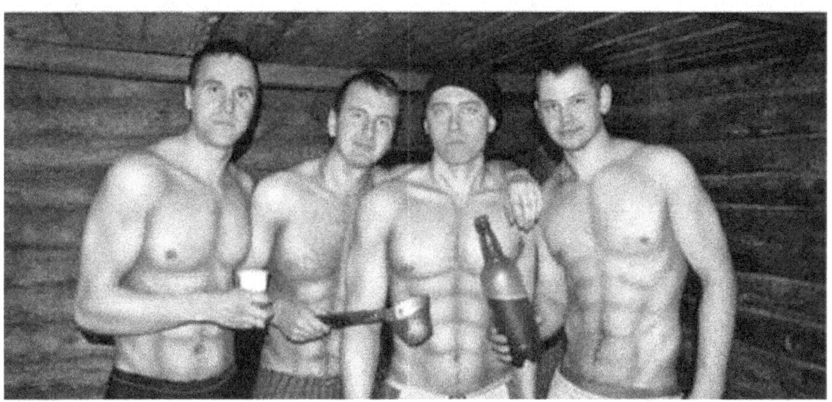

Magazines & TV adverts are selling you a scenario...

Just look what can be done with photo editing software.
[airbrushing]

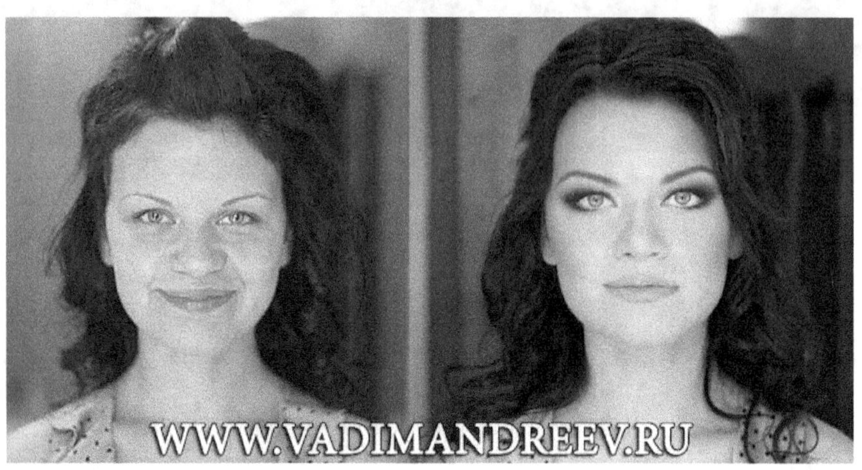

Clever stuff maybe but this is another example of unnecessary stress.

Continually looking at pictures of celebrities, happy families, new cars, designer clothes etc. is designed to make us all feel inadequate.

Check in with reality... You are great!

Now for the Good News!

Everything I've talked about is preventable & symptoms can be reversed

Prof Farid wrote [dailytelegraph.com.au 30 Nov 2011]

"Impossibly thin, tall, wrinkle-free and blemish-free models are routinely splashed onto billboards, advertisements, and magazine covers,"

He said these "highly idealised images have been linked to eating disorders and body image dissatisfaction in men, women, and children".

So the key here is find the best solution for you, take some small action steps and cut out the unnatural goals & lower your expectations...be realistic

Achieve something good for you

Homework

More baby steps...

- Start by asking yourself some challenging questions like... "Why am I overweight?", "How & when did the weight gain begin?", "What benefits will I gain when I achieve my goal?", & "How motivated & determined am I?" Listen to your own responses & work out why you are really holding onto the weight

-

- Say you would really like to lose 42 lbs or more...just think about losing 8lbs first & be pleased with yourself.#

-

- Have you got a pair of trousers or dress hanging in the cupboard that you can't wear at the moment? Dig them out & hang them where you can see them every day... Imagine going out in them, how you will feel

-

- Cut down on processed food

-

- Cut down on sugar – just make one commitment to yourself like never ever buying fizzy drinks again

Remember the compound effect...there is no rush!
Just do one thing at a time; turn one change into a new habit & then add the next one.

Go at your own pace & learn to feel great about your achievements.

Part III

Habit or addiction
Misreading hunger signals?
How to fool your body & kick start your metabolism
How to use EFT & acupressure
How to make your own Healthy Pot Noodle
Treat yourself to something nice

Habit v Addiction

You didn't get overweight overnight so you aren't going to
get back to your happy weight overnight

We've learned that we are not what we eat rather what we
assimilate i.e. what the body can actually use

Are you getting any nearer to identifying why you are
holding on to excess unnecessary weight?

By now I think you will be realising why dieting doesn't
work, that the answer isn't 'out there' the answer is within
you.

The science bit... when dopamine is released in the brain, we feel pleasure. When we eat things or do things that give us a surge of dopamine the desire to repeat the experience is very strong. The brain associates the behaviour with the sense of pleasure. We initially choose a behaviour but when it occurs repeatedly the behaviour moves from voluntary to automatic & voila a habit is formed

Addicted people talk about cravings because the brain has become accustomed to the substance or the pleasure & doesn't want to be without it.

To counter this we have to find a motivation for change, to weaken the habit & get rid of these self destructive patterns.

Hunger signals

The majority of us have never experienced real hunger. Hunger is a learned response; from childhood; we learn to please others by eating. Then it moves into a social activity, we eat with others & don't like to appear different

Sometimes it is a 'time of day' response... its lunchtime therefore I must be hungry

Dr. Darrell Wolfe says "Processed food offers little or no nutrition, but it has the taste people crave. Cravings are caused by of a lack of particular nutrients like minerals, vitamins, enzymes & good bacteria e.g. acidophilus. When we eat nourishing foods we supply the body with the right nutrients so it finds balance and turns off the hunger trigger; but when we eat processed, chemical-laden food the body is never satisfied because it gets so little nutrition."

Or maybe it is an emotional response... you are eating because you feel upset or depressed
I can tell that many of you will be resistant to these statements but I challenge you to try an experiment. You want to lose weight for you, for your own health & wellbeing? Then you are going to have to get out of your comfort zone occasionally.

When you get a craving & your hand reaches out ask yourself if you are hungry enough to eat a whole meal? Distraction techniques work as they put a gap between you, your subconscious mind & delay the gratification. Being sleep deprived also increases food cravings so when your hand reaches out try taking a 15 minute 'cat nap'.

Once a day for the next week at least I want you to do something totally different when you feel 'hungry'.

Say its 4 p.m. & you usually have a cup of tea & a snack... I want you to have a small drink of water & read a book, or go for a walk, or ring a friend... Anything but do what you normally do. Not only will you start to kick old habits you will begin to retrain your brain & gut responses.

Acupressure

An alternative traditional Chinese therapy well worth trying out is acupressure. This is where physical pressure is applied to acupuncture points on the body to clear blockages within the energy meridians.

There are several recognised acupressure points to stimulate parts of the body & mind to reduce addictions & reduce related anxiety.

First to try is the Shen Men point. Put your fingers behind your ears and your thumbs on the point & massage the point.

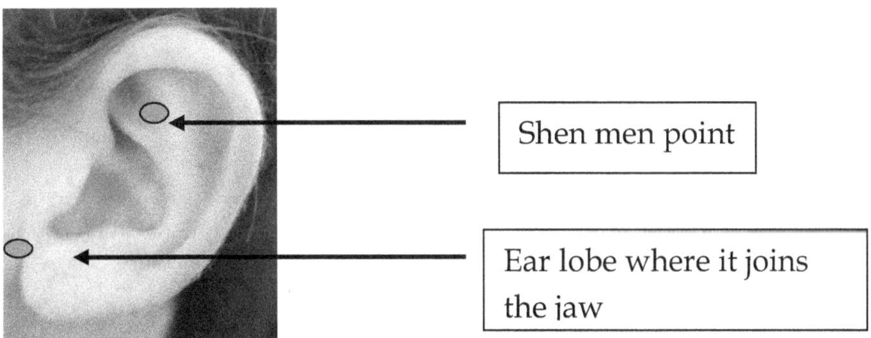

Or try massaging the ear lobe where it joins the jaw.

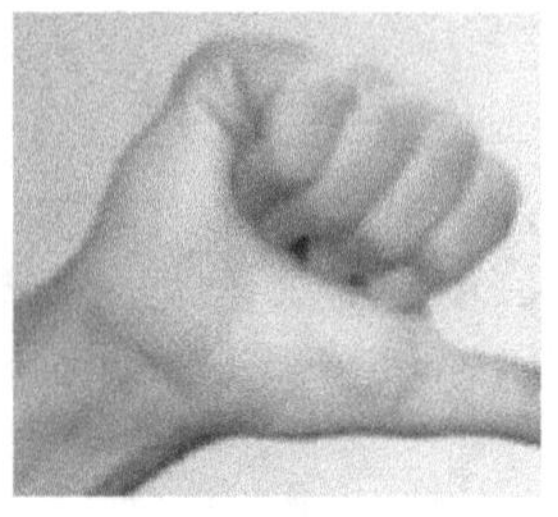

Or try putting your thumbs to your temples both sides of your head & then clench your back teeth together repeatedly noticing the movement in your temples.

When you get an 'eat now' signal try one of these for a few minutes. At the very least it will put a thinking gap in your subconscious mind so you start to reprogram & control your previous habits.

[Source: courtesy of Wikipedia & Acupressure.com]

Faster EFT

I am an EFT [Emotional Freedom Technique] Practitioner as well as a Hypnotherapist but I have found a new EFT method developed by Robert Smith gets results faster & doesn't take much time to learn. He has lots of videos on YouTube

It is basically just tapping in sequence on various acupressure points on the face and head for a few minutes. You might have heard of this before or might just think I'm crackers but please just try it out...I think you will be amazed

There are seven points we are going to use; top of head, between the eyebrows, side of the eye, under eye, two points on the chest and the wrist. To find the points on your chest feel down from your throat where there is a 'v' shape, move downwards & outwards below the collarbone until you come to a tender point when you press on it.

EFT technique

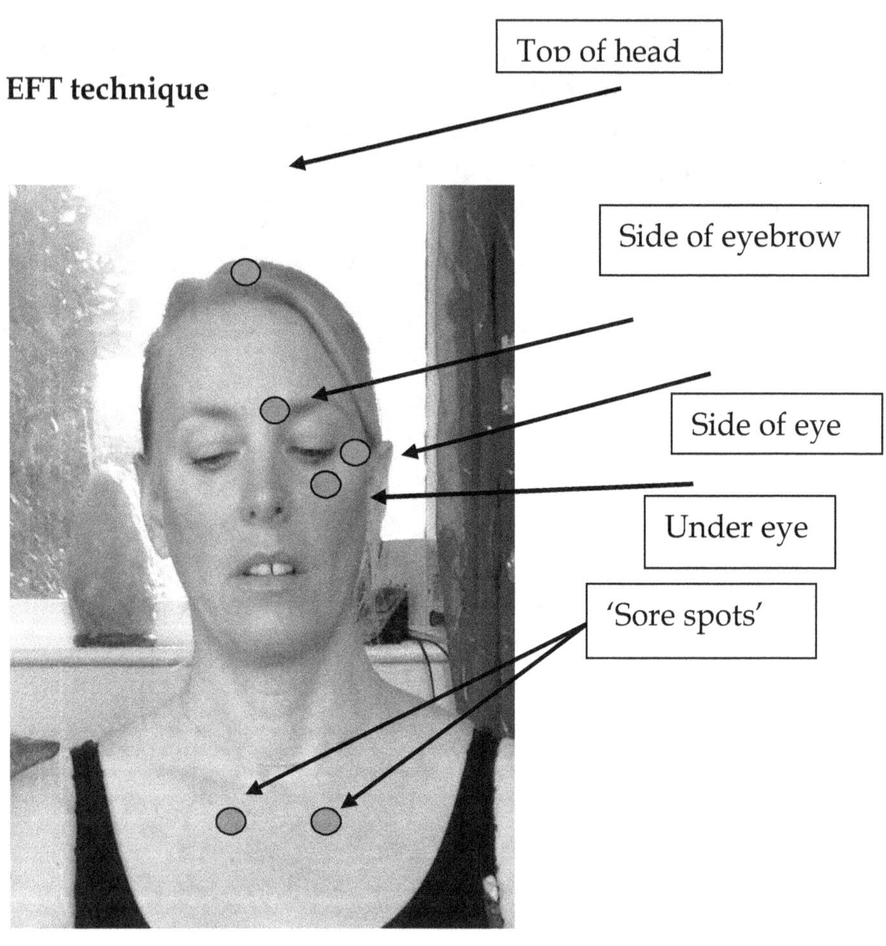

[This is my friend Lara who is a Dahn Yoga Teacher; she is also my model in my exercise book]

First concentrate on how you feel, on what the problem is &
then start tapping on each point 5 to 7 times

As you tap on each point in turn saying...

Top of head   Let it go
Side of eyebrow   Let it go
Side of eye   It's OK to let it go
Under eye   It's safe to let it go
Sore spots   Just let it go

Squeeze one wrist with the other hand, take a deep breath in
& blow it out ... say 'peace'

Recall a happy memory and enjoy it

Now go over the problem again and repeat the process

You can either do three rounds or just keeping tapping until
you feel you feel better about the problem
You could focus on addiction to sugar or sweets or whatever
you choose

Kick start Your Metabolism

What we've learned so far is that we are aiming to reprogram our subconscious mind to break our own vicious cycles & create new healthy habits.

1. Avoid insulin spikes so that your body uses its fat reserves rather than glucose.
2. Use EFT or acupressure to give you a longer gap between eating

Here are a few more ideas to help you:

Soup ... A liquidised meal lasts longer in the stomach than the same meal non-liquidised taken with a glass of water. The hormone, ghrelin is produced whenever the stomach is empty & tells us to eat. If we eat a vegetable soup it keeps us feeling full for approximately 1.5 hours longer - so to keep hunger at bay reduce the production of ghrelin ... because it also inhibits the breakdown of stored fat!

Eat more/weigh less: you can also fool your brain reactions by eating a huge meal of vegetables, salad, fruit, nuts & seeds smothered in apple cider vinegar, Himalayan salt, black pepper & olive oil. It will take a long time to eat, a long time to chew and a long time to digest. Smile & enjoy every mouthful.

Leave some food on the plate: I can hear the protests, but it's a good discipline....give it a try

Avoid 'fast food' & 'take-away' outlets they are often laced with addictive chemicals that switch off the hypothalamus

[see the book Fast Food Nation on my blog
www.susieellis.org/recommended-reading/]

How to Make Your Own Pot Noodle

Rather than eat all the nasty chemicals we can see on this label we can make our own version using proper food that our body can recognise & digest easily

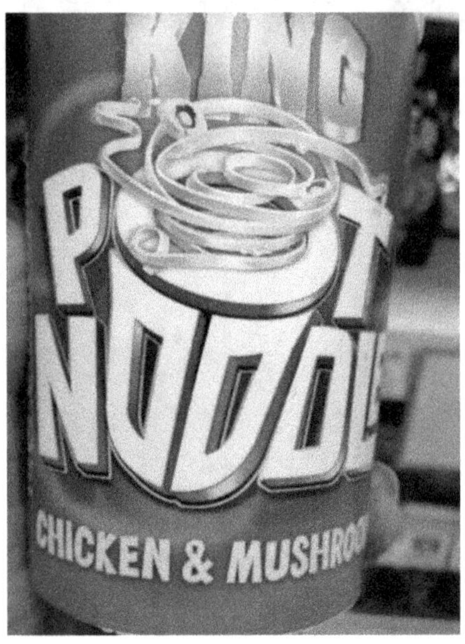

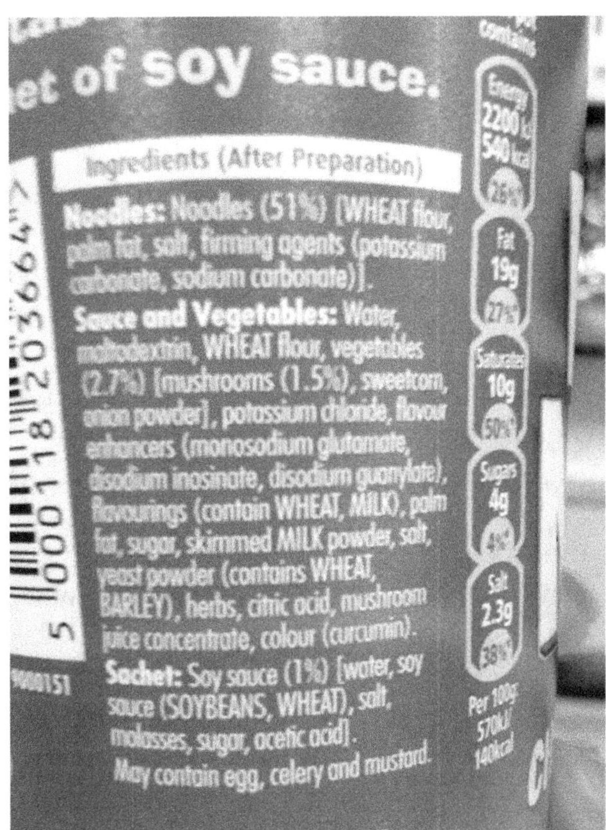

MSG and aspartame for instance, cross the blood-brain barrier and can do irreparable damage to the central nervous system

There isn't actually any chicken in this pot just flavouring!

51% noodles... only 2.7% vegetables & 1.5% mushrooms...

We can make a far better version

You can use fresh chopped vegetables cooked in stock, [or canned or frozen]
To be speedy use stock cubes but again read the label... some have additives in... there are also vegetarian stock cubes available and gluten free versions

Here is one idea: chop some mushrooms, onions, garlic & carrots into small dice, put in a saucepan with some frozen peas & simmer in vegetable stock for 5 minutes. Drain the vegetables through a sieve but keep the stock.

Put the noodles in the stock, bring to the boil turn off the heat & leave for 3 minutes.   Drain the noodles into a bowl, add the vegetables and as much stock as you like.

Rice noodles are good to use as they are also gluten free so this recipe can be adapted for everyone.

You can sprinkle with fermented soy sauce, salt & pepper or maybe some grated parmesan cheese.

The variations you can make are endless... Get your imagination going!

Homework

More baby steps...

- Three rounds of EFT every day
- Acupressure
- Write a list of foods you think you are addicted to
- Write a list of triggers & work out how & why the weight gain started
- Treat yourself to something nice

Remember the compound effect...there is no rush!
Just do one thing at a time; turn one change into a new habit
& then add the next one.
Go at your own pace & learn to feel great about your
achievements.

Part IV

Confidence

Putting my Hypnotherapist's 'hat' on, our nearest & dearest are often the most tricky when we start to make some positive changes... we have to recognise the signals and be ready to tackle them, after all this process is all about you and your progress, no-one else.

Other people's perception of you is none of your business... Be confident in the face of criticism & in your goals for YOU.

Our friends, family, work mates & acquaintances are all used to the way we are – that is their security. When you start to lose weight, get healthier & fitter you might run into some resistance. "oh you're lovely they way you are"... "Don't get too skinny it won't suit you"... "Wrinkles show up on thin people", "Oh come on you can have one more cake, it won't hurt" etc etc

When I hear people making remarks like that I wonder why
they are threatened & why they are voicing those particular
statements. Very often they are not up for making changes
in themselves for whatever reason & you stepping out of
their 'norm' makes <u>them</u> feel uncomfortable.

Just remember you are the important one! You are the one
who wants to be healthy & happy.

Find yourself a buddy with similar goals & join our
Facebook group where you can get all the support you need.

You can even book a Free 30 minutes Skype appointment
with me to help you get started...
https://www.susieellis.org/contact/

Hypothalamus

The hypothalamus is the portion of the brain that maintains internal balance or homeostasis. It controls body temperature, heart rate, blood pressure, appetite, body weight, hunger, thirst, metabolism, fatigue, influences the pituitary gland to release hormones, sleep and circadian rhythms

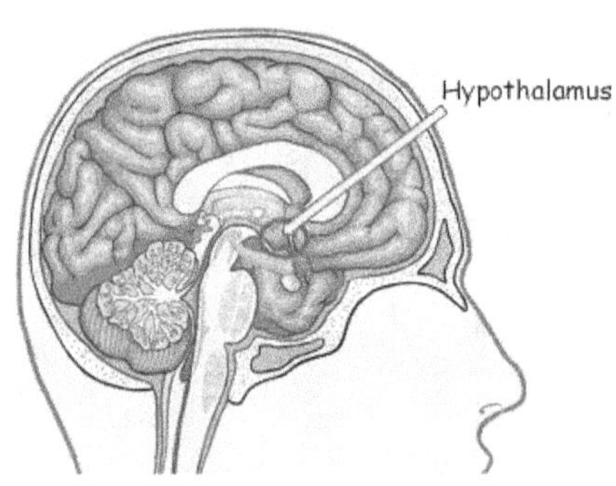

This tiny important part of our body is only about the size of an almond

The foods we eat form food memories in the brain so the key to keeping unwanted weight off is reprogramming the hypothalamus... & scientists are constantly working on it.

Obesity expert Louis Aronne, M.D., [I'm going to paraphrase as you don't need a lecture] says that eating a bad diet & overeating causes neurological damage. "Because of this damage, the signals don't get through about how much fat is stored. While some damage to the hypothalamus may be permanent, it's possible to reverse much of it."

Circadian Rhythm

This is the rhythm of life our bodies are designed to follow.
When this rhythm is interrupted it creates an extra stress
level which in turn can disrupt the digestive processes, sleep
cycle & more.

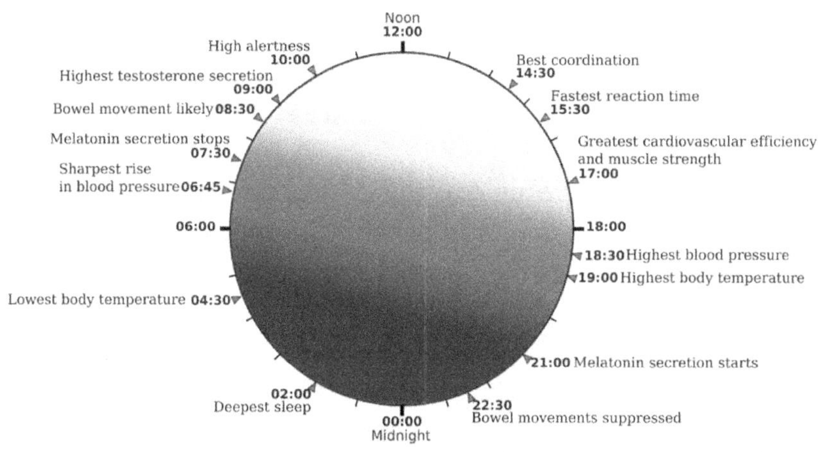

Photo courtesy of Lexarlighting.com

Shift workers are at a disadvantage as their circadian rhythm
is constantly being upset.

If you work from 19:00 to 07:00 for instance try & eat your
supper before going to work, lunch during your shift &
breakfast before going to bed & try to sleep between 09:00 &
17:00

Retrain the Brain

So.... how are we going to do that I hear you ask?

By overloading the body [& brain] with the foods it does understand - to desensitise it from stuff it has been fed until now.

There are lots of examples in this book ... like slow down whilst you are eating & give your hypothalamus time to kick in & tell you that you are full... it takes around 15 minutes

In the same article Louis Aronne, M.D., says that retooling your diet to be rich in health-promoting foods can stop and even reverse the damage done by an unhealthy one.

At the University of Liverpool, the researchers also looked at the impact of essential fatty acids, known to be beneficial to brain health... & sure enough, they appear to modulate some of the negative effects of saturated fats and carbohydrates.

This is why 'low fat' labels on food are a nonsense. It is the type of fat we need that is important. We need Omega 3, 6 & 9. We don't need Margarine, lard or hydrogenated fat & I will go into that in detail in the next part.

Mindfulness

Deepak Chopra says that we need to concentrate on what we eat & not do anything else... no TV, radio or music, no distractions; just focus on totally enjoying every mouthful. This calming focus aids digestion & assimilation.

Yoga & mindfulness practitioners suggest the same... by truly focussing on preparing & eating food we love to eat we slow down naturally and then only eat enough to feel full.

Never feel guilty about anything you put in your mouth... this is a back to front way of re programming your subconscious mind. You will begin to notice everything you are eating & question yourself about the necessity for eating something & if you really are enjoying it or if it is just a habit that you can be without.

Challenge Yourself

- Only cook enough for the meal you are about to eat so you are not tempted to eat leftovers. If you are bulk cooking separate the portions for freezing before you sit down to eat your meal.

- Leave something on the plate i.e. don't eat everything... eat slowly & tell yourself you are full & don't need any more.

- Crises usually occur around baby food & kids mealtimes... It is very tempting just to finish what they leave. Put smaller portions on their plates or bowls so they can't leave anything for you to pinch!

- Allow yourself to imagine how good it will feel as your clothes get looser; & when they are looser wear them with a belt so you can feel the difference

Cooking

Cooking from scratch v ready meals:

Some people find the concept of cooking from scratch daunting but if you can get your head around it, it really does help to heal your relationship with food. You begin to focus on what tastes good & the individual ingredients you are putting together rather than the act of just grabbing a ready meal out of the freezer & shoving it in the oven.

You can go one step further & good twice as much as you need & freeze half for another occasion... making your own ready meal for when you are short of time.

This saves money too... compare the cost & portion size of a home made a cottage pie to a supermarket version. I made 12 portions for £4.50, $7.16 which is around 38p or 60 cents each!

Buying in bulk & meal planning ahead for your week is really economical. You could also get together with a friend & swap dishes or donate a meal to a new mum or friend in need

Meal Ideas

Jacket potato ....or baked sweet potato or half a butternut squash

Served with:
Hummus, tomato salad & broccoli slaw...these can all be made a day ahead & kept in the 'fridge

To make hummus drain a carton of chickpeas & blend them with a chopped onion, 2 or 3 cloves of garlic, Himalayan salt, black pepper, lemon juice & olive oil. Taste & adjust seasoning

To make a basic tomato salad slice some tomatoes & onions. Chop a couple of cloves of garlic. Layer them alternately in a dish, season well & drizzle over apple cider vinegar or balsamic vinegar then pour over olive oil.

To make a broccoli slaw just chop the broccoli finely add grated carrot, chopped spring onions [scallions] & garlic. Place in a serving dish, season well & drizzle over apple cider vinegar or balsamic vinegar then pour over olive oil or hemp oil.

[all the ingredients nutritional value is improved by buying organic if possible]

Make two Freeze One

'Cottage' Pie   Serves 5/6

Peel & cut 500g swede [rutabaga] into large chunks

Wash 500 g potatoes & cut into same size chunks
Cook in boiling water for 10 minutes & leave to cool...

Put 1 tablespoon olive or coconut oil in a pan & gently fry 1
onion, 2 - 3 cloves of garlic & 2 carrots [all finely chopped]
for 5 – 10 minutes, then add 250g mushrooms [quartered] &
fry for another 5 minutes. Transfer all the vegetables to a
bowl.

In the same pan add 500g lamb mince & cook until brown
then tip off the fat & return the vegetables from the bowl to
the pan.

Add 1 carton / 400g of chopped tomatoes, some tomato
puree, Himalayan salt & black pepper to taste. You can also
add any herbs you like...

Simmer for 15 minutes adding a little water if it gets too dry.

Grate the cooled swede & potato into a bowl, drizzle over
olive oil, season well & mix together until well coated.

Tip the mince mixture into an ovenproof dish & top with the
swede & potato mix.

Put in a pre heated oven 180c /350f /Gas 4 for about 40/45 minutes.

You can use any minced meat or quorn for the filling & you can use any combination of vegetables for the topping e.g. sweet potatoes, celeriac, carrots

A meat free filling can be made by sautéing 1 chopped onion, 2 diced carrots, 1 or 2 sticks of celery chopped & 2 - 3 chopped cloves of garlic until soft & golden then add 250g sliced chestnut mushrooms & cook for another 5 minutes.

Meanwhile simmer 250g green or puy lentils for about 40 minutes until soft then drain and add to the sautéed vegetables.

Add 2 tablespoons tomato puree, salt & pepper, bay leaf & herbs to taste, then 500 ml water or vegetable stock & 100 ml of red wine [optional]

Movement & Exercise

I am not suggesting anyone buys a gym membership & goes there every day... baby steps, just move a bit more than you do now, every day.

Perhaps get off the bus or train one stop earlier on the way to or home from work & walk

Go swimming once a week

If you work by a computer get up walk around every 30 minutes

Run up the stairs instead of walking or taking a lift [elevator]

Really stretch first thing in the morning to get your lymph system moving. [It doesn't have a pump like the heart & we need to get it functioning to rid our bodies of accumulated toxins]

If you are chair bound you can still move your legs & arms, rotate your ankles & neck, rotate your shoulders and stretch as well as you can

Look out for my movement & exercise book... coming soon

Homework

More baby steps…

- Stop feeling guilty about <u>anything</u> you eat, enjoy every mouthful

- Smaller or larger plate size & concentrate on chewing everything well & slow down

- Cook some meals from scratch [bulk cook put in freezer]

- Move, stretch & exercise more than you do at the moment

- Treat yourself to something nice

Remember the compound effect…there is no rush!

Just do one thing at a time; turn one change into a new habit & then add the next one.

Go at your own pace & learn to feel great about your achievements.

Kirlian Photography

Vegetables

The following sequence illustrates how easily the energy force of a mushroom can be depleted.

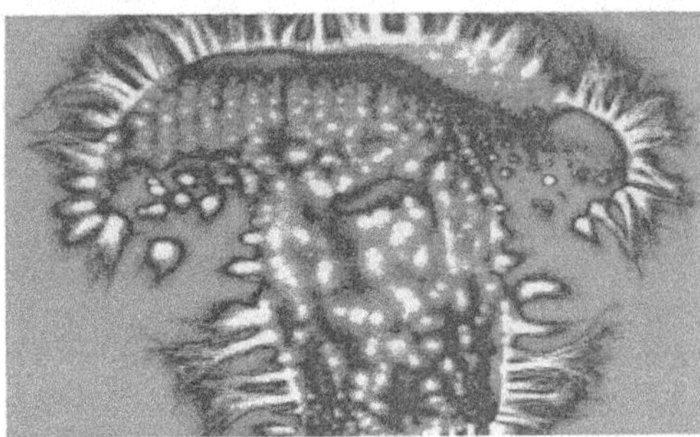

Organic mushroom.

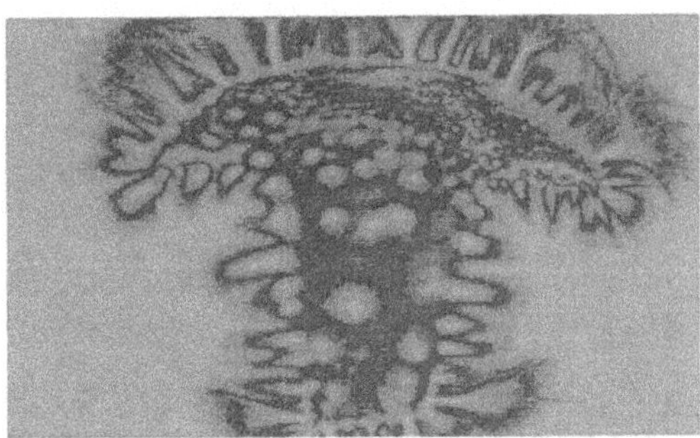

Non-organic mushroom showing less of an aura.

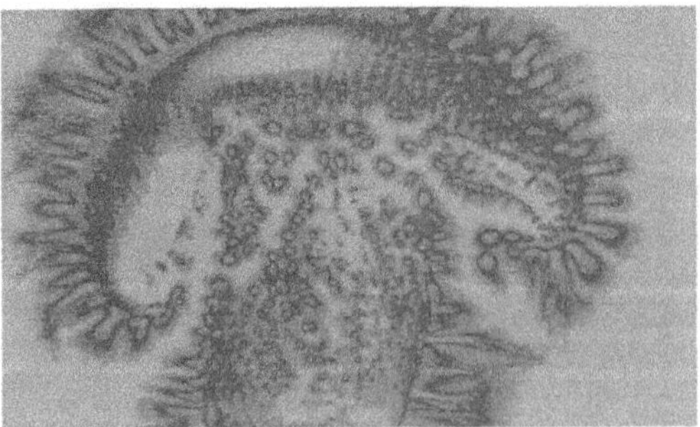

Non-organic mushroom lightly cooked but still retaining some of its life energy.

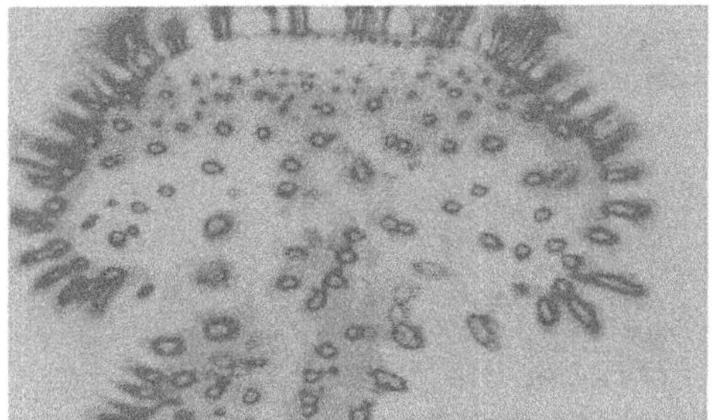

A sliced non-organic mushroom which has been left for 24 hours (not cooked) showing significant deterioration.

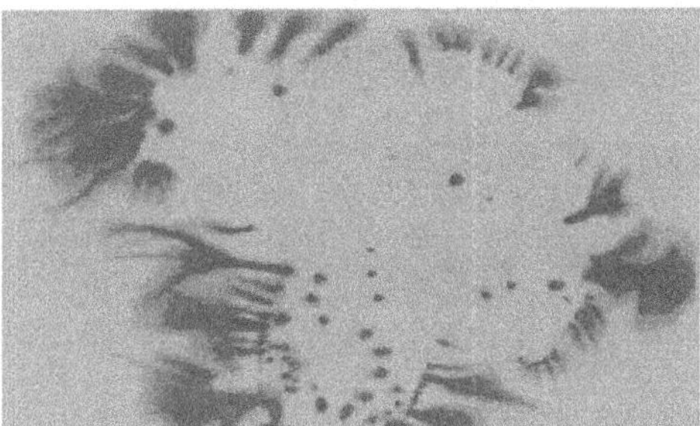

Finally, a micro-waved non-organic mushroom (5 seconds) is severely depleted of life energy.

Microwaved food

We highly recommend the *'What Doctors Don't Tell You' March 200 Vol. 10, No. 12 issue which spells out exactly the dangers of using micro wave ovens. The article covers: how micro waves work – the 'damning' German & Russian research – how food breaks down, losing its nutritional value – why convenience micro wave food is loaded with colouring and flavouring and the dangers of radiation.

Kirlian photography or electro photography is a brilliant tool to enable us to actually visualise the life force of the food we eat. The greater the life force the greater the nutritional value the better we assimilate the available nutrients

Microwaves

Day One — Pruned back
to record new growth
Microwaved Water
Purified Water
Day three
Microwaved Water
Purified Water
Day nine
Microwaved Water
Purified Water

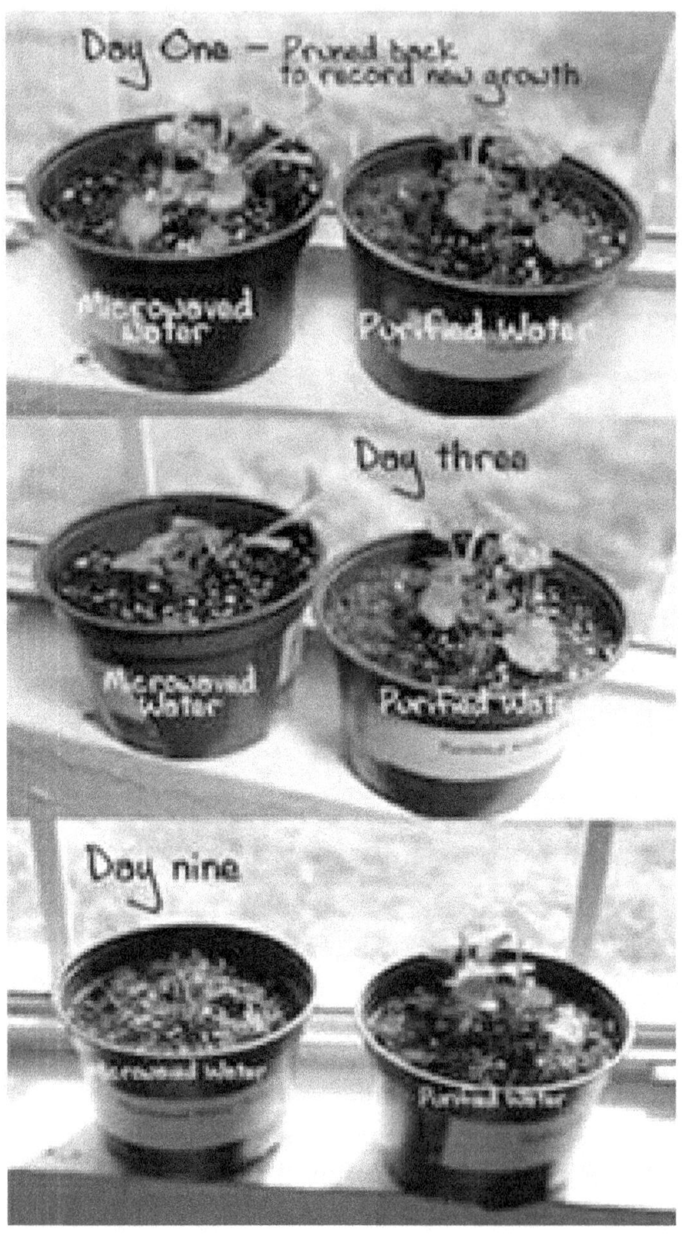

The kirlian photographs show clearly, & research supports the fact, that all nutritional value is wiped out so there is no point in eating microwaved food at all.

A high school experiment shows clearly that plants being given cold, previously microwaved water, die.

Personally I have never been happy with the thought of ingesting molecules that have been moving about & microwave ovens haven't been around long enough for a control study on our bodies...

Then there is the issue of toxic chemicals leaching out from the packaging... one woman died after being given a blood transfusion of microwaved blood in 1991....

& why is it recommended that we stand well away from a microwave often whilst it is switched on?

There is masses of information available for you to research & make up your own minds.

I never use one or eat food 'cooked' in one.

Intermittent Fasting

There has been quite a bit of discussion lately on Intermittent Fasting & the results are showing that it has a beneficial effect in reducing insulin resistance as it helps shift your body into burning fat rather than sugar & carbohydrates which in turn reduces the risk of chronic disease.

Dr Mercola suggests [28 /6/13] that to be effective you have to fast for 16 hours. Obviously you need to research & read all you can about it before even thinking of trying it out. I have actually been doing just that for years without realising until writing this... I was told that your body is still in elimination mode until noon. I just have fruit juice that I have squeezed myself.

You are probably horrified at the thought but you are most likely still in feast mode... the more you eat the more you want to eat.

It takes 6-8 hours for your body to metabolise glycogen & get to fat burning mode so the thinking is that if you are eating three meals a day plus snacks in between, your body is never able to catch up.

If you give your body space & time your cravings will diminish because it will get out of the habit of using sugar.

IF can also boost your level of HGH [human growth hormone] production by 1,200% to 2,000% which in turn speeds up your metabolism

Salt

Salt is essential for life, you cannot live without it. However there are enormous differences between the varieties of salt that are available to us to buy. These differences can have a major impact on your health.

Table salt is 97.5% sodium chloride and 2.5% chemicals [Ferro cyanide, talc, and silica aluminate are commonly included].

Sea salt used to be a good alternative but this is no longer the case. The oceans are becoming dumping grounds for toxic substances like mercury, PCBs & dioxins. Oil spills in the ocean are becoming more frequent and with 89% of sea salt producers now refining their salt; sea salt simply isn't as healthy as it used to be. Some people however, are fans of Celtic Sea salt so it is well worth you doing some research for yourself.

Looked at under a microscope you would see irregular and isolated crystalline structures disconnected from the natural elements surrounding them. This means that, however many vital minerals it may contain, they cannot be easily absorbed by the body without expending masses of energy. Your body's net gain is small compared to the loss of energy.

Mineral or rock salt is another alternative but the natural elements lack compression and are only attached to the surface and in the gaps in the crystalline structure.

Therefore your body cannot absorb or metabolise them.

However......the crystalline structure of crystal salt is not isolated from the 84 inherent mineral elements. This means that the energy content in the form of minerals can be easily absorbed and metabolised by the body. It has a vital energetic effect and your body gets an ample net gain with little energy loss.

Crystal salts from the Himalayas do not burden your body; it is the highest grade of salt; has a perfect crystalline structure; is immune to electromagnetic fields; and contains no environmental pollutants.

If you would like to read the whole article I have written on the subject of sale please get it touch & I will send it to you

Butter v Spreads

The debate rolls on... but yet again it is down to reading labels & eating food that the body understands how to process

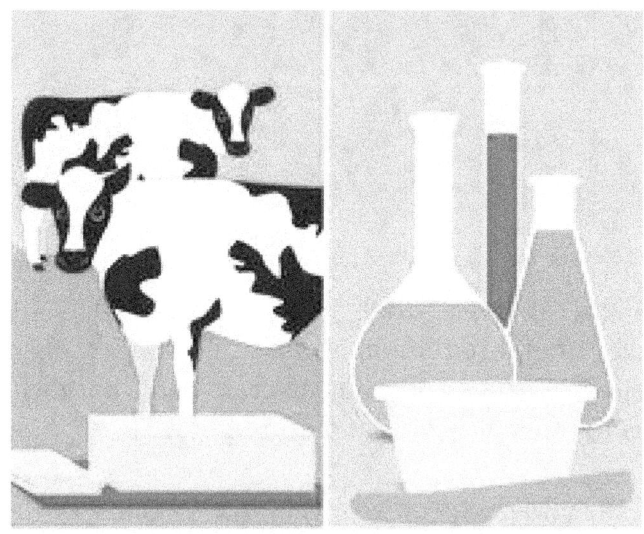

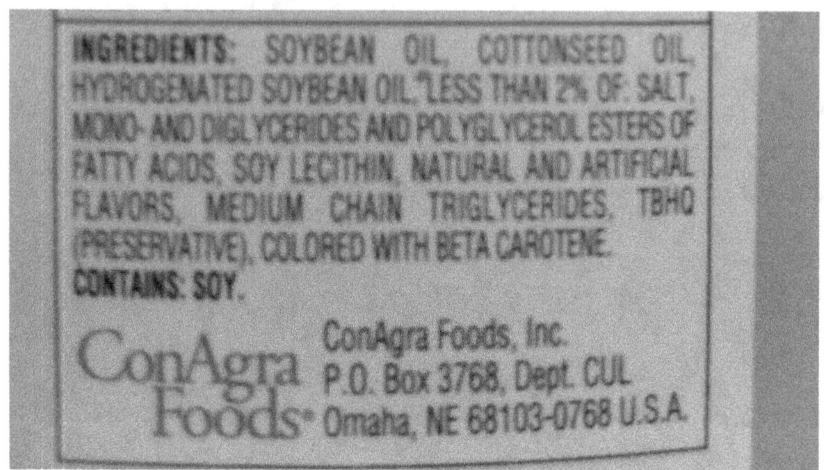

Photo courtesy of fearlesseating.net

An emulsifier manufacturer, palsgaard.com states "Aeration, crystallization, fat reduction and plastification: Control these four basic properties and you can craft your margarine products to meet almost any requirement." !

There is the GMO aspect, which I am especially keen to avoid, & then in processing the oils for margarine or spread the oils are heated to unnaturally high temperatures, & then treated with hexane & other solvents ... this is another instance of being sold to.

Butter can be made easily, put some milk in a jar with a lid & shake vigorously. Children often have fun doing this in schools as an experiment.

Benefits of Oil

As we touched on in Part IV, EFAs or essential fatty acids, omega 3 6 & 9 are, amongst other things, essential to reprogramming the brain, resetting the hypothalamus & lubricating joints.

Coconut oil is best used for cooking as it doesn't denature when heated & olive oil is best for drizzling over food. I am also a great fan of Hemp oil.

Olive Oil

Olive oil contains:
  * Oleic Acid, a monounsaturated omega-9 fatty acid [55%-83%]
  * Linoleic Acid, a polyunsaturated omega-6 fatty acid [3.5%-21%]
  * Palmitic Acid, a saturated fatty acid [7.5%-20%]
  * Stearic Acid, a saturated fatty acid [0.5%-5%]
  * Linolenic Acid/alpha-Linolenic Acid, a polyunsaturated omega-3 fatty acid[0.5%-1.5%]

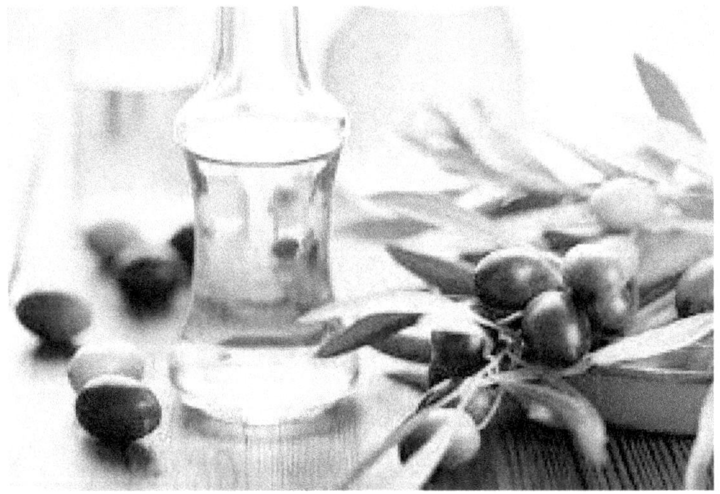

photo courtesy of oliveoilexcellence.com

The benefits of olive oil are extensive:

- Counters the effect of ageing: polyphenols, antioxidants, reverse oxidative damage
- Reduces the risk of coronary heart disease
- Increases the immune system
- Decreases inflammatory response
- Squalene and lignans : components being studied for their possible effects on cancer
- Lowers the levels of total blood cholesterol, LDL-cholesterol and triglycerides
- Rich in antioxidants, especially vitamin E
- Decreases both systolic and diastolic blood pressure
- Reduces the risk of type II diabetes
- Reduces levels of obesity
- Reduces the risk of metabolic syndrome [big belly syndrome, a combination of abdominal obesity, high blood pressure, abnormal cholesterol, and high blood sugar]
- Less likelihood of developing rheumatoid arthritis
- Improves bone mineralization and calcification
- Helps prevent the onset of Osteoporosis
- Protects from risk of stroke
- Reduces endothelial damage and dysfunction [ageing of the heart]
- Lowers the risk of depression & mental illness
- Contributes to the prevention of malignant melanoma [skin cancer]
- Oleocanthal reduces the risk of Alzheimer's & the cognitive decline
- Used for skincare since ancient times
- Massaging prevents sports injuries, relieves muscle fatigue, and eliminates lactic acid build up

- Contributes to the relief of seborrheic dermatitis, acne, psoriasis & atopic dermatitis
- Inhibits the growth of Staphylococcus aureus & Candida albicans
- Reduces the discomfort of haemorrhoids & anal fissures

NB: may be used in cooking but best eaten raw

Coconut oil

Coconut oil contains:
- Caprylic acid, a saturated fatty acid 9%
- Decanoic, a saturated fatty acid 10%
- Lauric, a saturated fatty acid 52%
- Myristic, a saturated fatty acid 19%
- Palmitic, a saturated fatty acid 11%
- Oleic, a monounsaturated fatty acid 8%

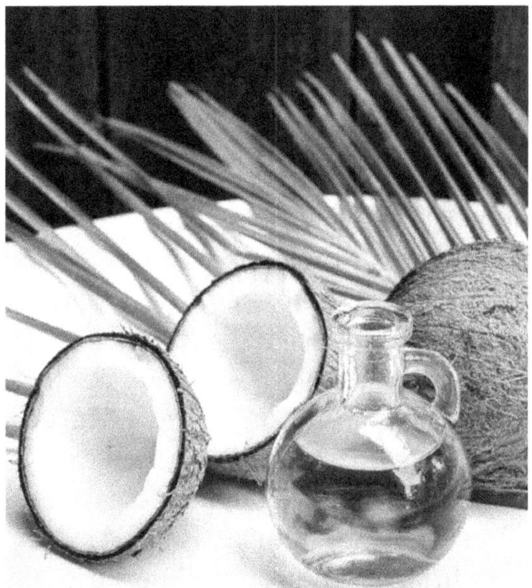

photo courtesy of coconut_oil-pulling.net

The benefits of Coconut oil:

- Many book & internet searches contain the huge number of benefits from using coconut oil from medicinal to skin care
- The medium-chain triglycerides (MCTs) in coconut oil can increase the metabolic rate, they go straight to the liver as a quick source of energy also having a therapeutic effect on disorders such as epilepsy & Alzheimer's
- Lauric acid & monolaurin can kill bacteria, viruses and fungi
- Reduces hunger
- Raises HDL, good, cholesterol and lowers the LDL, bad, cholesterol
- Improves blood coagulation & lipids reducing the risk of heart disease
- 60% of the diet of the people of Tokelau, an island in the South Pacific, is from coconuts/saturated fat & they have no evidence of heart disease.
- Decreases abdominal fat – a study of 40 obese women over 12 weeks taking 30ml a day reduced their BMI & waistline – a study of 20 obese men over 4 weeks showed an average waistline decrease of 2.86 cm
- Improves dry skin/ moisturiser
- Hair conditioner/re-growth / dandruff
- Effective as a sunscreen
- Make up remover
- Toothpaste
- Lip balm
- Deodorant

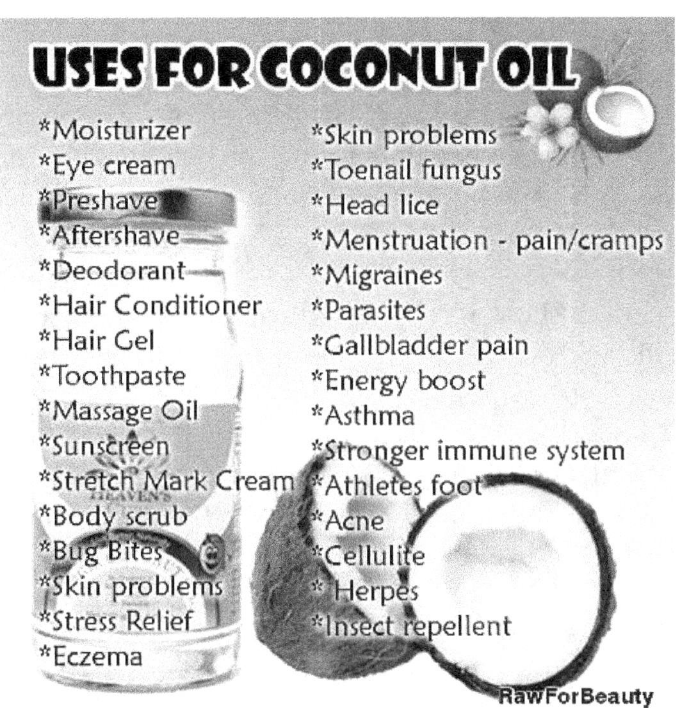

Oil pulling: Oral health is massively important to our immune system & gut health. Swish a spoonful around your teeth & gums for 5 minutes daily to begin with & increase to 15 minutes & spit out into a bin [not down the sink] This process removes toxins & bacteria.... then rinse your mouth with water or water with bicarbonate of soda or dissolved Himalayan salt water.

Hemp oil

According to a new study in the Journal of Agricultural and Food Chemistry researchers found the health promoting qualities of hemp oil include sterols, aliphatic alcohols and linolenic acids.

Sterols lower cholesterol and reduce the risk of heart attack. Linolenic acid [Omega-3] has been known to prevent coronary heart disease.

Aliphatic alcohols lower cholesterol & reduce 'sticky' blood... keeps the platelets moving. Phytol is an antioxidant & fights free radicals.

Tocopherol is beneficial against degenerative diseases like atherosclerosis & Alzheimer's.

Hemp seed oil is also beneficial for the skin & contains Vitamins A, C, D & beta carotene, plus minerals phosphorus, potassium, magnesium, sulphur & calcium.

Source: medicalnewstoday.com

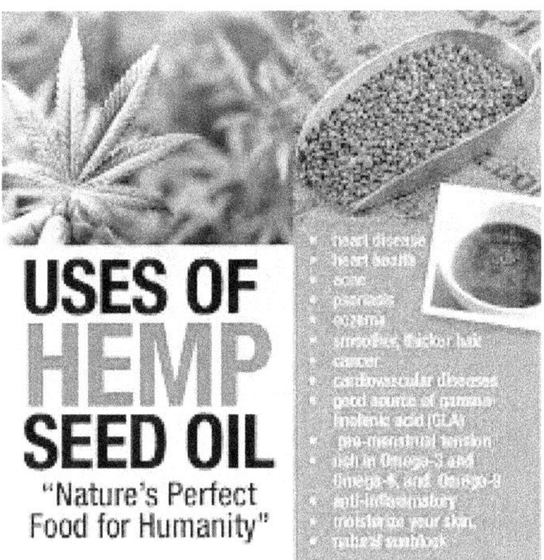

Photo courtesy of cryptonews.biz

Eczema: People with this condition do not have enough water in their skin cells so the imbalance of the regulation of skin shedding & water loss causes damage to the skin barrier.

Hemp oil hydrates the skin & maintains the functioning of this barrier. The fatty acids contain compounds resembling skin lipids [fats] so hemp oil penetrates the skin surface restoring its elasticity & reduces itching & inflammation. The beneficial effects are enhanced if also taken orally.

Source: oilypedia.com

NB: best not to be used for cooking

Water & Hydration

Drinking water when you first wake up has been linked to helping to cure & prevention of certain illnesses such as headaches, body aches, arthritis, heart problems, epilepsy, obesity, tuberculosis, meningitis, kidney disease, vomiting, gastritis, diabetes, constipation, uterine disease, ear and throat disease.

First thing in the morning before doing anything else, drink 1 litre of water. Start slowly with 1 glass & increase the quantity gradually over time.

Wait 45 minutes before eating or drinking anything; eat breakfast [or not if you are doing Intermittent Fasting] & then do not eat or drink anything for 2 hours.

Research shows that positive results will be seen, for example:
High blood Pressure - 30 days
Gastric Problems - 10 days
Diabetes - 30 days
Constipation - 10 days
Cancer -180 days

At mealtimes consider what you drink...cold water slows down the digestive process and solidifies oily foods. These solidified oils react with the stomach acid & they are absorbed quickly by the intestinal wall. Long-term accumulation of these digested oils can lead to serious illness. Perhaps it is worth considering drinking hot liquids with meals as the Chinese and Japanese do.

Source: naturalcuresnotmedicine.com

Soda & Alcohol

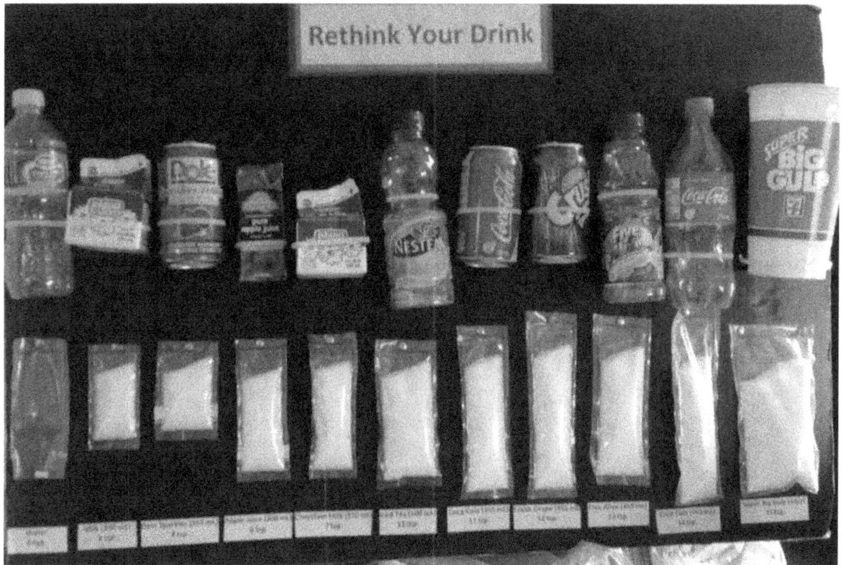

Photo Courtesy of Sustain our Africa

This was a school project... they must have had fun creating it

There's an amazing video circulating on YouTube of Jeremy Paxman interviewing one of the Directors of Coke & challenging him on the amount of sugar in the drink.... this vital information is now getting the publicity that is needed.

What he didn't address was the Phosphoric Acid content though. I suppose we ought to be grateful that cocaine was removed from the formula in 1903 ... 9 mg per glass!

There is also a proven link between regular cola intake & osteoporosis.

Katherine Tucker, PhD, associate professor of nutritional epidemiology at Tufts University, collected data on a total of 1,672 women and 1,148 men studied from 1996 to 2001. She said " the problem with cola is that you're getting those doses of phosphoric acid without any calcium. It's not balanced, and that extra phosphorus binds with calcium and prevents it from being absorbed."

Source: medscape.com

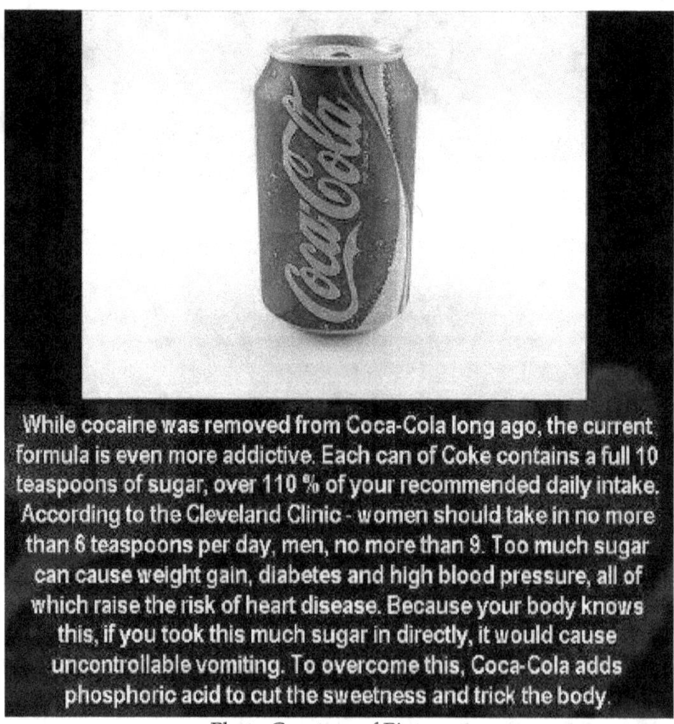

Photo Courtesy of Pinterest

Food for thought...

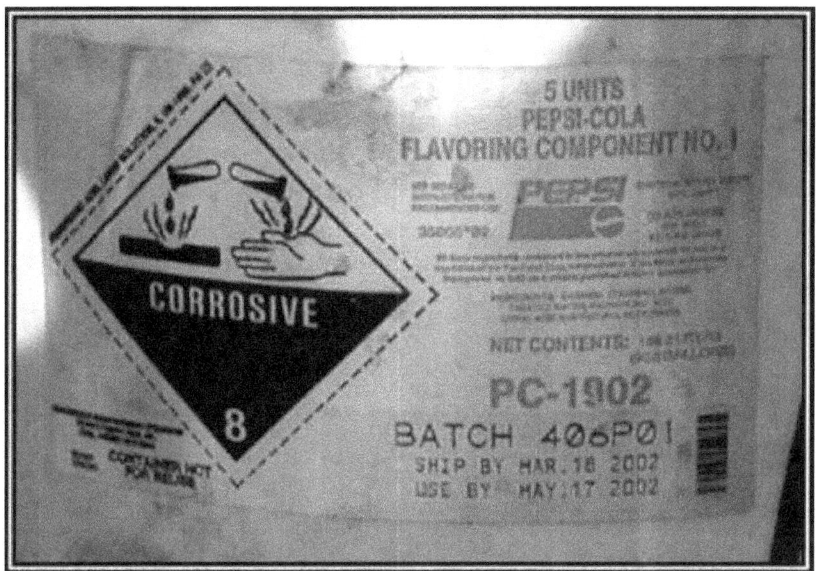

Source: Motivationals.org

ASPARTAME:

is the technical name for brand's like NutraSweet, Equal, Spoonful, and many others.
It is an artificial sweetener made from aspartic acid, used predominately as a sugar substitute.
It is currently in use **in over 6,000 products** that you may use everyday,
ranging from chewing gum and diet soda to prescription medications.
Aspartame was previously considered by the <u>**Department of Defense (DOD)**</u> as a potential **biological-warfare neurotoxin**.
Regardless of that fact, and after the FDA itself kept aspartame off the market for over 15 years, it later approved it
for dry goods in 1981 and then for carbonated beverages in 1983.

Symptoms:

chronic fatigue and immune deficiency syndrome, grand mal seizures, decreased vision, pain in eyes, ringing in ears, headache,
confusion, and <u>**DEATH**</u>. (Please read the **FDA's OWN list of 92 symptoms** for MANY more) Note: <u>**Five deaths were reported
prior to 1987, since then, figures have not been made public**</u>. According to the **FDA's own audit** on aspartame, the Bressler Report,
aspartame triggers **brain tumors, mammary tumors, pancreatic tumors, ovarian tumors, pituitary adenomas, uterine tumors,** etc.
Aspartame has also been shown to trigger **birth defects and miscarriages** - not just if the mother uses it, but the father also.

At temperatures of about 85 degrees, aspartame begins to break down into its base components.
These include: **methanol** (wood alcohol, known to street alcoholics as the alcohol that makes you go blind), <u>**formaldehyde** (a neurotoxin</u>
and embalming agent), **formic acid** (ant venom), and **diketopiperazine** (a known carcinogenic that causes brain tumors in animals).
Please note that the average human body temperature is 98.6 degrees.

Search Term: "Aspartame"
Do your own research, form your own conclusions.

Photo courtesy of livefreenatural.com

Think about your alcohol consumption...

Your liver burns alcohol rather than fat & contributes to belly fat

Calories in alcohol are 'empty calories' i.e. they have no nutritional value so in one way people who consume a lot of beer for instance are going to lose weight fast just by switching to a lower calorie beverage!

Alcohol stimulates your appetite & you might be full from a meal of the same amount of calories from food but several drinks might not fill you up. Research shows that if you drink before or during a meal, both your inhibitions and willpower are reduced.

Whilst drinking alcohol you are more likely to overeat, especially greasy or fried foods, which adds inches to your waistline. Try & delay drinking until you have finished your meal.

Alcohol is also a diuretic causing water loss and dehydration. Important minerals, such as magnesium, potassium, calcium and zinc are lost with the water.

Minerals are vital to the maintenance of all the organs of the body.

Good Ideas

- Shopping... Don't shop when you are hungry, there will be too many temptations

- Gradually replace processed foods with healthier choices as things in your kitchen store cupboard run out

- Green tea & apple cider vinegar boost metabolism

- Pasta with a tomato or vegetable sauce is far better than cream or meat sauces

- Eat a couple of vegetarian meals a week or more

- If you are having wine dilute it half & half with fizzy water

- Compare the calories in 'diet' food with other foods e.g. diet bars v ordinary biscuits

- Buy organic wherever possible

- If you need a snack have an apple & a few almonds or walnuts

- No more take away meals [or restrict them severely] – this will save your health & your bank balance

Recipes

Vegetable soup:

Slice some onions & garlic & fry on a low heat in coconut oil until opaque then add chopped vegetables e.g. carrots &peas, leek & potato.

Cover with water or vegetable stock & simmer until the vegetables are cooked.

Leave to cool for a bit & puree with a stick blender until smooth.

Add Himalayan salt & black pepper to taste & more liquid if needed to make the consistency you like best.

Seed & fruit balls:

In a food processor put a few apricots, figs & a tablespoon of pumpkin seeds & a tablespoon of sunflower seeds then pulse until the mixture gathers together in a ball.

Make small balls & put them in the 'fridge to set... a good supply of healthy treats [keep them covered as they take on other flavours]

Real food Ice Cream:

Bring 500ml double cream [organic] to the boil, add 3 ozs / 70g sugar [organic cane unbleached] & stir to dissolve.

Whisk 3 egg yolks [organic free range] & slowly whisk in the cream mixture.

Leave to cool & then pour the mixture through a sieve into a lidded container.

Freeze for at least 3 hours.

Variation: infuse a vanilla pod in the hot cream.

Remember you will need to take it out of the freezer well ahead of serving as it has no emulsifiers [plasticisers] in it

Now you have egg whites left over from the ice cream you can make your own chewy nut bars.

Chewy nut bars:
3 egg whites
10 ozs / 300g shredded coconut
10 ozs / 300g chopped nuts [substitute some of the weight with chopped dried apricots &/or figs]
2 fl ozs [3/4 tablespoons] local honey
1 tsp vanilla [opt]
pinch of unrefined sea salt

Preheat oven to 325 F, 170 C, Gas 5 and line a baking sheet with parchment paper.

In a large bowl, whisk together egg whites, honey, sea salt and vanilla.

Add the coconut, nuts & fruit and mix with your hands until well combined. [Wet your hands with cold water to prevent sticking]

Make little mounds (about 2 tsp.) and place them on the baking sheet. [approx 20]

Bake in the oven until the edges of the cookie are golden (for about 10-15 minutes).

Leave to cool on a wire rack

Healthy Popcorn:
Heat a saucepan & put in a handful of popping corn [GMO free] put the lid on the pan & shake the pan occasionally. You will hear the popping... Eat just as it is or sprinkle with Himalayan salt.

Healthy Chocolate: Mix coconut oil with equal parts cacao powder and honey for a natural chocolate sauce, or allow it to set in the fridge in an ice cube tray for healthy homemade chocolates.

Homework

- Ditch the microwave

- Use butter instead of spread

- Invest in some coconut oil for cooking and olive oil for drizzling

- Drink more water... 1 glass when you wake up

- Ban soda [fizzy drinks] from your life

& remember the compound effect...there is no rush.

Just do one thing at a time; turn one change into a new habit & then add the next one.

Go at your own pace & learn to feel great about your achievements.

Coming Next:

Look out for…

- My follow up emails to keep in touch

- Join us & get support at our Facebook group " Susie's Health & Weight loss Mastermind"
https://www.facebook.com/groups/SusiesMastermindCoaching/

- Movement & Exercise programme

- 10 Steps Recipe book

- Clear out & Detox

- Fermented food & Probiotics

- Tough love intense programme

- Sleep & Obesity

- Free calorie PDF

- Free article on Salt

About the Author

I'm Susie Ellis mother of four, a
business & lifestyle coach & a qualified
Hypnotherapist. Over the years I have
become more & more interested in
maintaining a healthy lifestyle, not
having to worry about my weight &
avoiding pharmaceuticals.

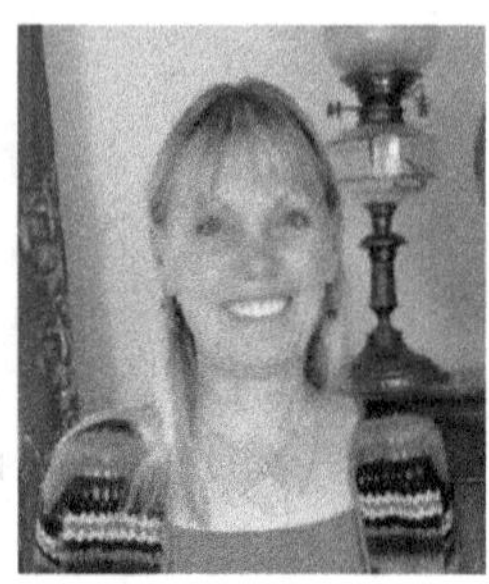

My mother was a yoyo dieter so I learned first-hand, at an
early age, that this was an addiction. I didn't have a weight
problem but I gained one through circumstance. I even took
some amphetamines, supposedly to speed up my
metabolism, as a teenager, but fortunately I collapsed,
stopped taking them & vowed never to go down that route
again. Keeping fit & drinking water wasn't on my family's
agenda.

Having had a lifelong interest in food & it's affects on health;
plus one of my children being cured of 'hyperactivity
syndrome' by dietary changes, I have been encouraged to
learn the truth, help others & share my ideas with the world.

Many people have asked me for help losing weight & eating
a healthier way but, long term, often found it so hard that
they gave up.

Game for the ultimate challenge I began to explore &
research how I could help people lose weight, be healthier,
boost their immune systems & maintain their ideal body
image forever. This book & programme is the result.

Disclaimer

The entire contents of this book & related programme are based solely upon the opinions & views of the author unless otherwise noted. Individual articles are based upon the opinions of the respective author, who retains copyright as marked. The information in this book, programme & website is not intended to replace a one to one relationship with a qualified health care professional and is not intended as medical advice.   It is intended as a sharing of knowledge and information from the research and experience of Susie Ellis and the wider community.

9 781797 568065